Contradicting Maternity

Contradicting Maternity

HIV-positive motherhood in South Africa

Carol Long

Wits University Press
1 Jan Smuts Avenue
Johannesburg
South Africa
http://witspress.wits.ac.za

First published 2009

The publishers gratefully acknowledge financial support for this
publication from the Faculty of the Humanities, University of the
Witwatersrand, Johannesburg.

ISBN 978-1-86814-494-5

Photographs on pages 8, 9, 11, 14-18 copyright © Gideon Mendel
and on pages 12 and 13 copyright © James Nachtwey

Cover artwork: *Thula Mama* by Karen Lilje
Cover design and layout by Hybridesign
Printed and bound by Creda Communications

Contents

Acknowledgements
vi

Preface by Juliet Mitchell
vii

1. Introduction
1

2. Facing the HIV-positive Mother
23

3. The Joys of Motherhood
54

4. Finding the HIV-positive Mother
81

5. Minding Baby's Body
105

6. Mother's Mind
127

7. Mother's Body
145

8. *Thula Mama*
168

9. Contradicting Maternity
190

Appendix : Interview Content
209

Bibliography
211

Index
229

Acknowledgements

I would like to thank the mothers who generously shared their experiences with me and whose stories are told in this book. Thanks to the hospital for their humane and dedicated service despite the odds. Special thanks to Juliet Mitchell, who took me under her wing and guided me through this project with brilliance and compassion. To my family, particularly my parents Linda and Nigel, and to my dear friends who supported me through this process, I could not have done it without you. And to Michael, of course ...

Sincere appreciation to the Faculty of Humanities, University of the Witwatersrand, Johannesburg, for financial support and provision of an intellectual environment. Within the Faculty, the School of Human and Community Development has provided an intellectual home.

I would also like to thank the bodies who funded my PhD, upon which this book is based, including the Ernest Oppenheimer Memorial Trust, the Skye Foundation, the Cambridge Commonwealth Trust and the Smuts Memorial Fund.

Finally, thank you to the staff at Wits University Press, including Melanie Pequeux and Veronica Klipp, for making this book a beautifully presented reality.

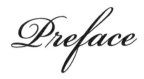
Preface

One cold white day in Cambridge, England, Carol Long, an always shivering and very blonde young woman, told me she wanted to research the experience of being simultaneously given a death and life sentence. She proposed to interview women diagnosed pregnant and HIV positive at the very same moment; the test for pregnancy revealing the disease. Instantly my stomach contracted in identification with the unknown mother, but almost immediately, as Carol talked on and I questioned, I realised how very little I understood. My gratitude for the journey Carol took us on will always be immense.

The modest presentation of a central part of this journey here in book form is extremely welcome; the book captures the work's importance. The importance is, of course, practical – aspects of policy, of psychological and political understanding can be re-thought: for instance, I was struck by the importance of community. The mothers talked to Carol and to each other in their hospital groups and medical check-ups – a stigmatised disease lived in social isolation and the privacy of the home changes somewhat by being shared, its pariah status slightly eroded. But beyond the implications for how to change attitudes and therefore the conditions of both HIV and motherhood, what I want to convey is a larger, more general sense of why this book truly matters.

It matters of course enormously to all the women for whom the mothers of this book speak. We, the readers, are almost certainly not these women; but, for all our sakes, we need to listen. If we do not, our 'cultural anaesthesia' will prevail: our knowledge of what Carol Long has heard as she asked and listened to the world's catastrophes and its people's trauma, will be without meaning. A meaningless knowledge diminishes us all. Instead of this *Contradicting Maternity* breaks through this anaesthesia, eroding the binaries of pain and pleasure, fear and joy, even death and life, us and them. It collapses our categories: the objects of research have become the subjects who address us with their big loves and small hates, with their lives and their impending deaths, their children's heritage.

Professor J C W Mitchell
Cambridge University, UK

1. Introduction

HIV prevalence among South African women attending antenatal clinics is estimated at 30.2 per cent: i.e. nearly one in three pregnant mothers is HIV-positive (Department of Health, 2006). Because this is also the time when women are particularly motivated to test, many discover that they are HIV-positive only when they realise that they are pregnant. Hearing that one is pregnant may produce a variety of emotions and responses. Whether excited or scared or devastated, it is news that changes one's life. In a context in which motherhood is highly valued, there is always recourse to the expectation that one will be admired by others and will experience joy and fulfilment. Hearing that one is HIV-positive produces very different kinds of emotions and expectations, particularly in an environment that is saturated by misunderstanding and horror at the social category of 'HIV-positive'. The process of becoming both a mother and HIV-positive begins in the moment when the news is received, but proceeds through a series of confusions, prejudices and adjustments in which the process of becoming exists in an uneasy space between internal reality and external discourses. In this sense, it is transitional and paradoxical, with opportunity for painful splits.

This means that HIV-positive mothers enter into two contradictory identities simultaneously: the denigrated, abject and feared identity of being HIV-positive and the idealised identity of motherhood, with all its associations of purity and goodness. Both identities hold complex and competing personal and social meanings, with motherhood and HIV invoking powerful discursive positions. Both motherhood and HIV are created in a moment of intimate sexual contact, but both exist uneasily with sexuality. Motherhood, paradoxically, is associated with chastity rather than sexuality, exemplified in the archetypal Virgin Mary (Kristeva, 1986; Warner, 1976). HIV becomes a metaphor for aberrant sexuality, whether justified or not (Sontag, 1988).

Being diagnosed HIV-positive when one is pregnant means entering into these two contradictory identities, which independently hold complex meanings of loss and gain, creativity and destructiveness, and which collide in the same moment in time. Motherhood is the ultimate act of creativity, in which life is given form. The miracle of life, however, is reminiscent of the nearness of death (Pines, 1997); creating another being evokes fears of destructiveness directed towards something so helpless (Parker, 1995); while the gain of motherhood also involves loss of identity in the service of motherhood (Oakley, 1980), as well as fears of the loss of one's child. HIV evokes very different associations of creativity and destructiveness. Something has been created in one's body that is trying to destroy one. This directly evokes the oppositions of life and death, particularly because outward signs of the virus cannot be seen for a potentially significant period of time before serious illness sets in. Questions of what one is to accomplish in one's life, as well as how one is going to die – universal questions that most of us spend a fair amount of time avoiding – become more urgent with an HIV-positive diagnosis. These questions take on a particular quality in relation to the social significations of HIV; to morality, death and abjection; and to calls to 'live positively'. With the promise of antiretroviral medication, the progression of the virus can be retarded, which may make a significant difference to one's health. However, in the inner world where fear is as important as reality, the existence of the virus inside one's body encourages one to contemplate death. In the social world of discursive meanings, an HIV-positive diagnosis is responded to with prejudice and rejection, regardless of how healthy or unhealthy one is.

Becoming an HIV-positive mother means that these opposites meet one another within one person, evoking love and hate, tragedy and joy, fear and hope simultaneously. HIV-positive motherhood also causes uncertainty regarding one's own identity, one's future and the future of one's baby. Because HIV can possibly (but not probably) be transmitted from mother to child, uncertainty regarding whether one will transmit HIV to one's child provides fertile and perilous soil for fantasy. This uncertainty occurs in the context of dominant discourses of motherhood that posit that the baby is all-important; the mother not at all. Making sense of oneself as a mother – for one's baby, but also for oneself – means negotiating the strong emotional resonances of HIV-positive motherhood through very powerful and socially sanctioned discourses of both motherhood and HIV.

This uneasy existence of HIV-positive motherhood between these two wildly differing extremes may be part of the reason for the discomfort the HIV-positive mother provokes in the popular and scientific imagination. There seems to be a sense that, within the urgency of the HIV pandemic, HIV-positive mothers are not terribly important – or, at least, not as important as their children – or as women who, still innocent, are not yet infected. This is borne out in the available literature on HIV-positive motherhood. The few books that have been written are biographical in nature and concern an individual mother and/or her child. This is strikingly reflected in the personal and emotive titles of these books. Writing about HIV-positive motherhood in this genre implies a painfully individual experience – *one* mother isolated with her child or children and with her tragedy and triumph. The small body of empirical literature that studies HIV-positive mothers, in contrast, seems to be obsessed with the implicit assumption that HIV-positive mothers must be *bad* mothers, with a lack of attention to HIV-positive motherhood as a category in its own right. Mothers are usually only of interest insofar as they pose a risk to children and family. Focusing on the well-being of children poses a danger that the mother fades out of focus and becomes seen only as a vehicle for her baby's well-being.

Given the stigma that many HIV-positive mothers experience, this book resists these morally evaluative questions. It explores mothers' experiences of themselves as HIV-positive, and as mothers imagining themselves from their children's perspectives and from their own perspectives. The decision to shift focus to the mother is as much a political choice as one informed by the paucity of knowledge about HIV-positive motherhood. The book explores maternal experience by focusing on the stories of real women. It is based on interviews conducted with black South African mothers diagnosed as HIV-positive when pregnant.[1] Pregnant women and new mothers who attended an HIV clinic in Johannesburg were invited to volunteer to take part in individual interviews exploring their experiences of being HIV-positive and of motherhood. The interviews started with the question, 'What has the experience been like for you?' and, although I had a specific series of questions in mind, from that initial question on the interviews largely went wherever it was important for participants to take them. The interview content is included in the appendix to this book. In all, 110 interviews were conducted with 50 women. Some women chose to participate in a single interview, while others attended between two and seven interviews. All the women were invited to participate in multiple interviews depending upon what felt comfortable for them. Some participants were counsellors at the clinic, and these interviews formed a backdrop for the analysis. The opportunity to conduct a large number of interviews, as well as the richness and sophistication with which women brought their experiences into the interviews, has been invaluable in understanding the nuances of HIV-positive motherhood from the subjectivity of mothers themselves. It also became clear that the category 'HIV-positive mother' is a fiction: while motherhood was regularly coloured by HIV and

1   I am using 'black' as a political category to include coloured and Indian; i.e., in the modern parlance, all 'previously disadvantaged' women. I mostly interviewed black African women, but there were also coloured and Indian women, as well as one white woman, whom I excluded from the analysis because her story was quite different (and very racialised).

produced particular concerns and ways of interacting with children, it did not produce a particular brand of motherhood, and there were as many differences in mothering as there were similarities.[2]

The presentation of women's stories in this book draws on the traditions of discourse analysis and psychoanalysis. Discourse analysis provides a method for analysing the ways in which subjects and objects are constructed within power relations and through broader social meanings. Psychoanalysis offers ways of reading fantasies, conflicts, anxieties and desires and of foregrounding layers of affect. It should be noted, however, that the intention is not to 'psychoanalyse', individualise or pathologise, but rather to trace the interactions between psychodynamic and discursive processes in the negotiation of motherhood and HIV status in order to understand the contradictory subject positions held. A primary aim of *Contradicting Maternity* is to convey a rich sense of the experience of being an HIV-positive mother. To this end, it has been important to conjure up the lives and imaginations of the women who participated in this study without constructing them as irrevocably 'other'. Relying heavily on stories and quotations, the book aims to convey a thick description of the experiences and preoccupations of HIV-positive mothers in relation to their sexuality, their relationships, their bodies, their babies and their own maternal perspectives.

IMAGES OF HIV-POSITIVE MOTHERHOOD

A central argument of the book is that maternal HIV-positive experience is more complex than the caricatures presented in the public and scientific imagination, and that it is important to understand HIV-positive motherhood from the mother's perspective, and not just from the more seductive and socially sanctioned perspective of her child. One way

2   This book is specifically concerned with HIV-positive motherhood and focuses on interview material related to this. Other primary issues related to gender, heterosexuality and the HIV-positive body are reported elsewhere (see Long, 2006; Long, forthcoming).

of thinking about the social imagination of HIV-positive motherhood is through images of HIV-positive mothers. When I came upon the photographs presented below through contemplating the disjunctions between social discourses and lived experiences of HIV-infected maternity, my first response to the photographs was of both familiarity and shock, since they were so patently about human suffering. Images contextualise, because 'seeing comes before words' (Berger, 1972: 7). Photographs give the reader faces and environments that cannot be conveyed in words.

As I examined the photographs further, however, it became clear that this is not all photographs do. They also objectify, exploit, distance and victimise (Berger, 1972; Sontag, 2003). They create a disturbance of ownership, transforming subject into object, owned now by the photographer and the onlooker (Barthes, 1980). This is perhaps particularly the case when one regards the pain of others (Sontag, 2003), a genre of photography that has become almost synonymous with 'art'. The more gruesome the photograph, the more 'serious' the photographer. In this sense, photographs decontextualise. As Barthes (1980: 90) puts it, a photograph 'is without culture: when it is painful, nothing in it can transform grief into mourning'.

As Sontag (2003) struggles against her earlier ideas (Sontag, 1979) that such photographs exploit and sap our capacity to respond meaningfully to the pain of others, she comes upon a similar political dilemma. Are such photographs good or bad? Do they create empathy or apathy? Should they be upheld as showing us what we should know or should they be critiqued for turning human suffering into a masquerade? It seems that she does not entirely settle these dilemmas. For example, much of her essay is critical, but it ends with praise for photographs dealing with the pain of others, because they remind us that we do not understand. Of particular relevance to the photographs under discussion here, she also leaves the political implications unsettled:

The more remote or exotic the place, the more likely we are to have full frontal views of the dead and dying. Thus postcolonial Africa exists in the consciousness of the general public in the rich world ...

mainly as a succession of unforgettable photographs of large-eyed victims … [including] of whole families of indigent villagers dying of AIDS. These sights carry a *double message*. They show a suffering that is outrageous, unjust, and should be repaired. They confirm that this is the sort of thing that happens in that place. The ubiquity of those photographs, and those horrors, cannot help but nourish belief in the inevitability of tragedy in the benighted or backward – that is, poor – parts of the world (Sontag, 2003: 63–64; emphasis added).

The photographs chosen for presentation here are largely from highly acclaimed photographers whose explicit motivation is always to provoke awareness and empathy. Shock is used to promote a realisation of the severity of the epidemic. Outwardly, then, they aim to portray the first side of Sontag's 'double message', showing the outrageousness of suffering. They have achieved fame (and publication), however, in the developed world, and cannot escape its obverse: as Sontag says, they potentially 'confirm that this is the sort of thing that happens in … the benighted or backward – that is, poor – parts of the world'. The majority of photographs depicting AIDS in Africa fall into two broad categories, either portraying graphic images of suffering, often of emaciated bodies; or showing people's pride and defiance in response to the epidemic. In both categories, there are many faces, whether sick and hopeless; sad and mournful; or joyful, loving or defiant in the face of prejudice.

However, the more I examined the photographs, the more I noticed how consistently mothers were portrayed differently to 'people' and how infection seemed to be written differently in the presentation of their bodies. Although the focus of this study is not on the analysis of media images, I have found it useful to consider these photographs, because of their powerful portrayal of the HIV-positive mother in the public imagination. Interpretations offered for each photograph are partial, focusing on what the photograph may tell us about constructions of HIV-positive motherhood, but there is no claim of an 'authoritative' interpretation, and the reader is invited to reinterpret them according to his/her own understanding.

It is not entirely true that 'harrowing photographs do not inevitably lose their power to shock. But they are not much help if the task is to understand' (Sontag, 2003: 80). These photographs can therefore problematise the way in which HIV-positive motherhood is constructed. Whether intended by the photographer or not, the ways in which the 'HIV-positive mother' is portrayed, and the fact that she is often portrayed differently, bring some kind of understanding of the anxieties that this figure evokes and the social discourses in which she is located.

For example, Gideon Mendel's photo essay on AIDS in South Africa (Mendel, 2002), published in *The Guardian*, aims to portray the human faces and stories behind the appalling statistics. Like many other AIDS photographers, Mendel captures the tragedy of AIDS, but he also explicitly aims to convey the multiple faces of the pandemic, including those of hope, courage and laughter, and of the tenacity of those speaking out in

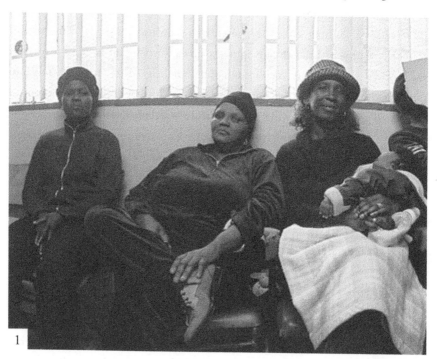

1

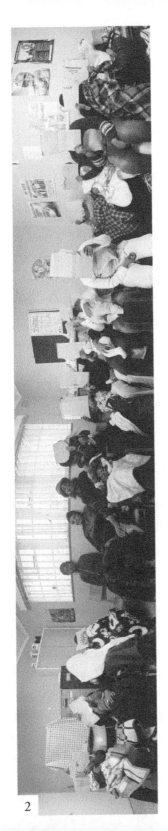

his photographs against the prejudice associated with the pandemic. He presents photographs of a variety of people in different situations. When visiting his website, one sees among these a photograph (photograph 1) of three women, one holding her baby, and reads the caption: 'Why can't they give us the treatment to make the mother healthy because who is going to look after that negative child if we are gone?'

By clicking on the photograph, the viewer enters the antenatal clinic where these women are sitting (photograph 2).

When viewed in its context, the photograph is no longer about HIV-positive mothers defiantly speaking out. On the contrary, amid the many faces and voices in the essay, the mothers, hiding behind their hospital files, are silent and hidden. Their facelessness is noticeable, evoking the shame of being HIV-positive mothers. This shame is counterposed against the familiar slogan, 'Be wise condomize', on the wall, which advice, the composition implies, these women clearly did not follow, their pregnant bodies proof of their irresponsible sexuality.

The mother in photograph 3, from Mendel's collection, is also hidden, this time behind a hot-water bottle. The focal point of the photograph is her thin and presumably HIV-positive child. The foregrounding of the child's thin body leads one to imagine both shame and guilt: the mother is responsible for her child's infection. She is sad and ashamed, but she is also damaging or destructive. Attention is detracted away from the reflection in the mirror. Even at the margins of the photograph, even in reflection, the mother's face cannot see and cannot be seen.

James Nachtwey (2001), whose photo essay in *Time* provoked debate about its graphic depictions of the horror of AIDS and its inclusion of emaciated bodies, includes a group of photographs united by the theme of motherhood and childhood. The mother's body is not at all emaciated: it is not present at all. Instead, the mother is represented in her absence, either replaced by images of caretakers holding children or by images of abandoned orphans or street children living in abject circumstances as a result, it is implied, of maternal HIV. It seems that motherhood

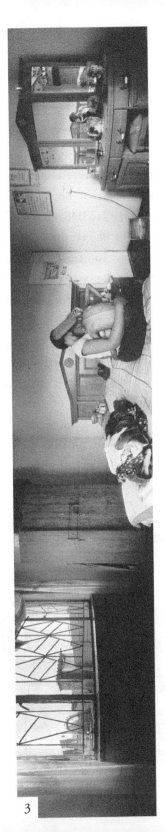

is shocking enough without the need for emaciated maternal bodies – there are very few such images to be found across the collections. Two photographs from Nachtwey's collection indicate her threat.

In the first (photograph 4), grandmother and grandchild gaze unhappily into the distance. We are told that both have AIDS. The photograph comments on the coexistence of AIDS independently contracted within families, portraying the pathos of grandmother and child, who obviously contracted HIV from different sources. The absence of the mother (the viewer is likely to imagine that she is dead, since the grandmother is caring for her child) directs sympathy towards the child and leaves the mother only insinuated as the source of infection. The mother is present in the form of her opposite: the Virgin Mary tending to the baby Jesus in the picture on the wall exemplifies the pinnacle of motherhood. The photograph presents us with categories of innocence: the child, the caring grandmother and the good mother who is an asexual virgin. The photograph is typically silent on the father, the other partner in infection. He is present only in the form of Joseph in the picture on the wall, possibly the most ineffectual father in history; the father figure, but not the real father.

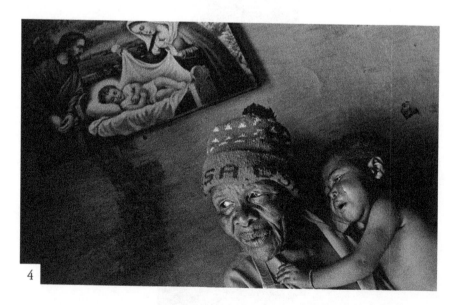

4

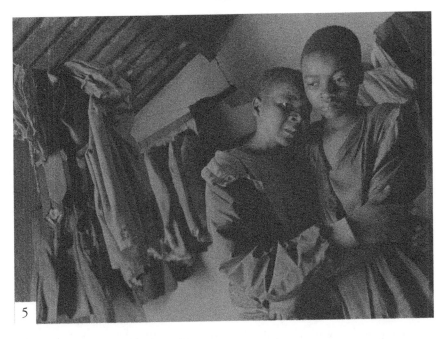

5

The actual mother is present in the next photograph (photograph 5) as a person rather than as a representation. The caption reads: 'A mother of several children (left) was afflicted by AIDS and had to be taken care of by one of her daughters, who consequently could no longer attend school.' The photograph confronts us with the tragedy of AIDS-related illness. Set in a domestic scene, it brings us closer to the struggles of everyday life. It also tells us a story about mothers and children: we are told that the mother has 'several children', and that the young woman in the photograph is one of those children. Here the threat is not only of infection, but of reproductivity, implied in the caption as irresponsibly endless. This procreative threat, it is implied, is also destructive, not only to the mother herself, but also to her daughter, who has been obliged to give up her schooling – and therefore her future – in order to care for her mother. It is unclear who the subject of the photograph is, the sick mother or the deprived daughter, but the photograph seems to imply the recursivity of the threat of maternal infection and its invasion of the subjecthood of her child.

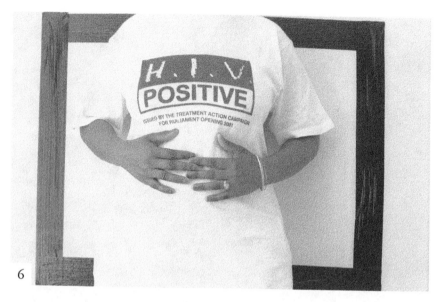

6

Photograph 6 is from a collection by Gideon Mendel entitled 'Looking AIDS in the face' and this photograph reflects a familiar theme in which 'looking AIDS in the face' often involves looking at faceless bodies. This person chose to be photographed with her hands at the focal point 'as a symbol of her renewed capacity to do her domestic chores'. The photograph is thus about activity and a renewed sense of agency in the world. It overtly draws attention to her hands, but covertly draws our attention to what her hands embrace: her tummy. The caption accompanying her photograph tells us something more about this tummy: she had previously been pregnant and her child, born prematurely, died at three months, around the same time that she discovered she was HIV-positive. The photograph is therefore ostensibly about her hands, but the traces of her tummy, and the sense of the proximity of procreation and destruction that is evoked, transform our understanding of the image.

The 'Looking AIDS in the face' collection is distinct in two ways. Firstly, those photographed were free to choose how they would like to represent themselves (hence the frame in the background), thereby taking some ownership over the form of representation. Secondly,

[u]nlike much ... other work done on the issue of HIV/AIDS in Africa, there are no images of sick and dying people here. The people photographed are dynamic and empowered. The haunting power of this work lies in the fact that while most of the images are gentle, the traumatic and painful material is contained within the text (Mendel, 2006: 43).

This collection aims, therefore, not to shock or to re-present, but to reflect images as chosen by those being photographed. Within this collection, there is a series of photographs in which mothers chose to represent their maternal presence, but also their maternal facelessness. Mother and baby are positioned in different configurations, but each photograph foregrounds the innocent child in contrast to the faceless mother.

In photograph 7, the baby shields the mother's face and the mother shields her baby from the camera. It is almost as if they are sharing a private moment. The caption tells us that the mother chose this frame because her baby had just tested HIV-negative. Despite this joyful news, the baby hides the mother's identity.

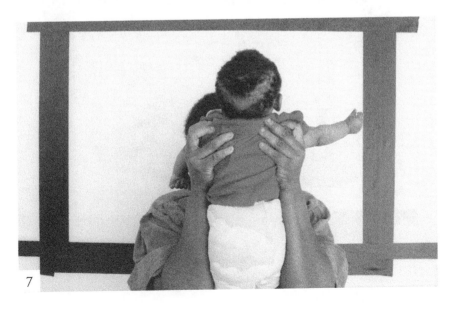

7

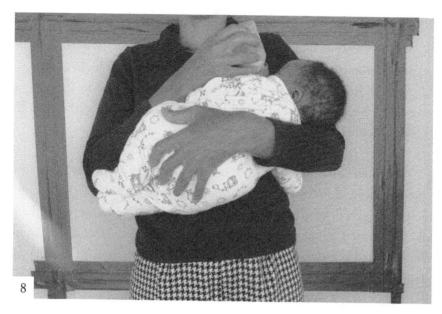

8

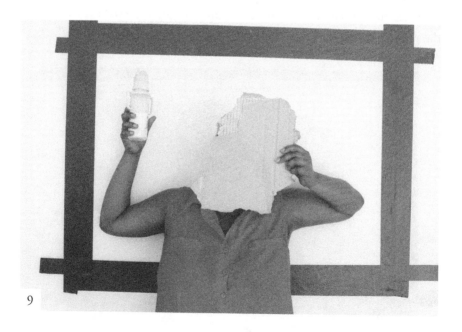

9

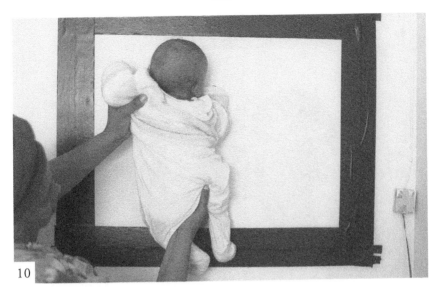

10

The mothers in photographs 8 and 9 both chose to represent their choice to bottle feed rather than breastfeed their babies in order to minimise the risk of HIV transmission. In both cases, the image is about the baby. The women hide their faces so as to avoid recognition, and also because their faces are less important than the bottle and the primary subject, the child.

Photograph 10 offers a similar representation of the centrality of the child and marginality of the mother. This particular mother is waiting for her baby to be old enough to be tested and is therefore unsure of her baby's status. It is this issue that is, for her, centre frame.

In contrast to images of facelessness, absence and destructiveness, photograph 11 presents a different image of the HIV-positive mother. This mother and her baby are both HIV-positive, but she has decided to represent an intimate moment between herself and her baby. Unusually, both her face and her joy are visible. She has refused to be represented as tragic, destructive or absent. The composition of the photograph also suggests the possibility of a maternal position in which the mother is the subject of the photograph: the child's face is somewhat blurred, with the effect that the mother is centre frame.

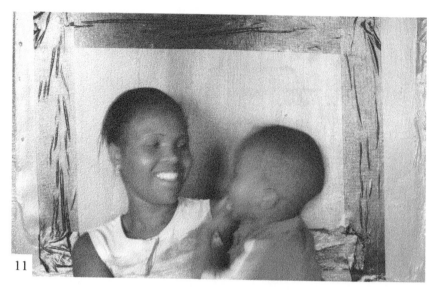

11

My telling of these images is from the point of view of my search for the mother within them; it provides one possible account in order to suggest that it is difficult for the idea of the HIV-positive mother to enter into the social world except through fantasies of abjection, infection, absence, blame and guilt. Around the edges of her body lurks dangerous sexuality, but not, ironically, a gendered relationship. The images do not portray fathers. Men are largely absent, despite their crucial role in the family drama of HIV/AIDS. Of course, these portrayals capture the seriousness and tragedy of HIV infection, as well as the desire to hide one's face; but, I would suggest, they also capture the fear and horror of public images of HIV-positive motherhood, fear and horror that belongs more squarely in the imagination of the onlooker than in the totality of the HIV-positive mother. The final image (photograph 11), but perhaps also the peripheries of the other images, suggests a different way of imagining and a different area of maternal imagination, and it is this multiplicity of maternity that this book will aim to explore.

ABOUT THIS BOOK

Contradicting Maternity can be read in different ways, and the book has different purposes. One purpose is to present a theoretical understanding, based on interview data, of motherhood in the context of HIV. This aspect of the book will appeal to academic readers. The second purpose of the book, which will appeal to both academic and non-academic readers, is to explore the stories of real mothers, aiming to preserve the complexity, sophistication, conflicts and joys expressed by them. The reader will therefore notice that there are two different styles in the book, which reflect these different nuances. Certain chapters foreground the theoretical voice, while others foreground the voices of the mothers themselves, although all the chapters are interested in both foregrounding and theorising maternal experience. In the chapters more centrally concerned with the mothers themselves, theoretical concerns are deliberately implicit so as not to detract from the importance of the mothers' voices.

There are also different perspectives in this book: those of the mothers and my own. Because I am writing the book, the mothers' voices are necessarily filtered through my own positioning as a white women, an academic and a clinical psychologist, as well as through the voices of the theories upon which I draw. My presentation of motherhood in the context of HIV is interpretive, although it is grounded heavily in the actual words of the mothers I interviewed. I experienced an ongoing debate about how much of myself to put in the book. For example, there were points in interviews where my own responses to the stories I was hearing were striking: points at which I was unable to hear something, or found myself uncharacteristically sympathetic or annoyed, sometimes wanting to adopt mothers or their babies, sometimes wishing I were somewhere else. I sometimes wondered why it might be, for example, that, at one point in an interview with a particular woman, I could not think of a single question to ask, even though this had not occurred before, or where I identified or disidentified with interviewees. I found it useful to note my internal responses during the process of writing in relation to the meanings I was writing about (e.g. the points in analysis where I felt stuck, or where I felt that meaning was proliferating out of control, or where I dreaded writing about a particular issue). Another relationship useful to reflect upon while writing concerned aesthetics. I often had to wonder whether my desire for beautiful words was working towards my desire to convey the sophistication and complexity of interview material or whether it was working to defend myself against some of the difficulty and ugliness of HIV-positive motherhood.

My initial intention was to write these experiences fully into the analysis. However, I was concerned about the extent to which these reflections would rewrite interview material in ways that distanced the experiences I was trying to convey. While it is important to state one's position, jokes about post-modern research (where it is all about the researcher) prompt caution about the practice of reflexivity. It could be argued that an overemphasis on the position of the researcher runs the risk of both reifying difference and detracting from the voices of interviewees. It is important to acknowledge that analysis is informed by my own subjectivity, but the inclusion of particular examples does not necessarily help to understand maternal experience and potentially complicates interpretation rather than making it more transparent. I have therefore limited reflections on my own position in the book, and have aimed to practise reflexivity by inserting my subjectivity into my writing, i.e. in a less descriptive and more process-oriented manner. I have used relationships with a trained psychoanalyst, who supervised the project, and with colleagues (including fellow graduate students, academics and clinical psychologists) to explore the analysis with the help of other subjectivities. This has provided a countercheck regarding the coherence of interpretation and the verity of its links to the data (Elliott, Fischer & Rennie, 1999; Taylor, 2001). Because the study has an unusually large sample size for qualitative research, it has also been easier to use repetitions in the data in order to reflect upon my interpretations.

Readers will also encounter the book through their own subjectivity and may read the accounts of mothers in different ways to the ones presented

INTRODUCTION

in this book. Each reader will find his/her own way to read the book, and I have deliberately avoided presenting a monolithic account. As one of the anonymous reviewers for the book favourably noted, *Contradicting Maternity* 'insists on complicating matters, rather than simplifying them. As such, it perhaps raises more questions than it answers'. Such questions invite possibilities for dialogue and for avoiding constricted understandings of motherhood in the context of HIV.

Overview of the book

Chapter 2, 'Facing the HIV-positive Mother', begins the book with an introduction to some of the women who participated in the study. After describing the context of the study, the stories of four women are introduced. The book deliberately begins with the stories of real mothers so as to highlight the complexity of their stories from the outset.

Chapter 3, 'The Joys of Motherhood', offers a critical interpretation of academic literature on motherhood, including feminist, psychodynamic and South African perspectives. It is hoped that consideration of motherhood as an identity, whether or not overshadowed by HIV, will encourage readers to encounter HIV-positive motherhood as a particular instance of motherhood, which, because of its extremity, allows us to examine identities of motherhood more broadly as well. Chapter 4, 'Finding the HIV-positive Mother', extends examination of the literature specifically in relation to HIV-positive motherhood. By reading this literature with a psychodynamic and discursive eye, some of the discomforts and assumptions of HIV-positive motherhood begin to emerge. This analysis argues that such studies are almost exclusively interested in the potential of mothers to damage their children. Like listening for slips of the tongue, I argue that one can read such studies with an eye to gaps and points of irrationality in order to understand the specific anxieties that the figure of the HIV-positive mother evokes in the scientific imagination. Specific themes of absence, death, guilt and abnormality are explored. This task leads into the second half of the chapter, in which discursive and psychodynamic frameworks, central to the theoretical framework of the book, are explored.

Chapters 5 to 8 present an analysis of interviews conducted with HIV-positive mothers. Chapters 5 and 6 focus on the maternal position in which the baby is the primary subject. Chapter 5, 'Minding Baby's Body', explores mothers' interactions with their babies' bodies and the ways in which they keep their babies' bodies in their own minds. Babies' bodies are encountered through the imaginations and fantasies of mothers, with the promise of medicine guiding, but not completely allaying, their fears. Chapter 6, 'Mother's Mind', explores the mother–infant relationship and maternal care, including breastfeeding, in order to suggest that maternal care has a particular quality in relation to HIV-positive motherhood, where maternal selflessness and the threat of HIV occupy centre stage.

Chapters 7 and 8 focus on the more marginal, but ever-present position of the mother herself, in which mothers foregrounded their own subjectivity *as mothers*, and from their own perspectives. Chapter 7, 'Mother's Body', asks where the mother's body, in contrast to the baby's body of previous chapters, is brought into interviews. The focus is on how maternal bodies are written into subjectivities of motherhood. Chapter 8, '*Thula Mama*', presents an analysis of the mother's voice, i.e. the ways in which mothers expressed their own loves, losses, tragedies and joys. It will be argued that the baby is the primary subject of the mother's attention, while the mother's own active position, from her own point of view, is secondary. Nonetheless, the active subjectivity of the mother is strikingly present, if not dominant. However, the mutual exclusivity between primary baby and secondary mother, so often implied by discourses of motherhood (e.g. good selfless mother versus bad selfish mother) cannot account for the interconnectedness of mother and baby in maternal subjectivity.

The book concludes with chapter 9, 'Contradicting Maternity', in which a synthesis of the book and a theoretical discussion of its implications for HIV-positive maternal subjectivity are explored.

2. Facing the HIV-positive Mother

In comparing the HIV-positive mother depicted in photographs and constructed in the literature (see chapter 4) to the women I interviewed, perhaps the most striking feature is that these images do not begin to convey the multiplicity or complexity of experiences of motherhood in the context of HIV infection. To construct a discrete and measurable object called the 'HIV-positive mother' is thus an impossible task. There were as many differences among women as there were similarities. This is further complicated by the fact that each woman had a different life story, which inflected her experience of motherhood in the context of HIV differently. It becomes clear that trying to characterise the HIV-positive mother implies that a type exists that is either productive of or produced by HIV infection – that either a certain type of person contracts HIV or that HIV invokes a certain brand of motherhood. The multiplicity of experience reflected in interviews with HIV-positive mothers implies that this unifying assumption is a form of monolithic stigmatisation.

The complexity of experience reflected in the data seems to further undercut the polarised descriptions implicit in the literature. Responses to the experience of motherhood raised a plethora of different issues. These issues were often entangled with one another, and were sometimes clearly defined and sometimes fragmented and disjointed; sometimes clearly articulable and sometimes inhabiting a space that went beyond what could be said. While the women spoke more fully and directly about the experience of being HIV-infected, discussion of motherhood had a much more contingent and shifting texture in interviews. It was easier for the women to talk about their HIV infection than it was to talk about themselves as mothers. This reflects the slipperiness of the concept of motherhood in broader psychological theory and public understanding of what it means to be a mother. Similarly, the experience of being HIV-positive, while easier for the women to talk about than experiences of motherhood, and, as the analysis will show, often talked about drawing on established and practised discourses, was nonetheless expressed in multiple ways. A positive diagnosis held different meanings in relation to different aspects of their lives and at different points in the telling: the experience of being HIV-positive was sometimes strange and exotic (echoing the object of the 'HIV-positive mother' in the scientific and popular imagination); sometimes all-eclipsing; and sometimes just another aspect, albeit an important and painful one, of everyday life.

This chapter places the women in this study within the ethos of the research setting and of their environment in order to contextualise some of the everyday 'realities' for black women living with HIV in South Africa. Because HIV circulates so powerfully in the social world and in its power relations and institutions, personal meanings and stories cannot be alienated from these social meanings. Conversely, an understanding of HIV-positive subjectivity cannot take subjectivity prior to HIV-diagnosis as a pre-existing and unmarked given, but as constituted within a particular social, economic and historical context. Furthermore, the image of the 'black HIV-positive mother' is one that potentially incites the imagination, offering easy flights of fancy aided by race, gender, ideals of motherhood and fantasies of HIV.

This leads to the second task of this chapter: to describe the context of women I interviewed in order to disrupt the homogeneity often implicit in the category of 'HIV-positive mother' and to unsettle the exoticism often associated with African women (Mama, 1995; Zivi, 1998). HIV-positive women are largely portrayed in public policy, through medical discourse and in popular culture as either unidimensional victims or as hazardous sources of infection, but seldom simply as women (Squire, 1993). Hogan (1998: 169) suggests that black women are othered in multiple ways by AIDS discourse, which compounds existing racial discrimination:

> When poor women and women of colour are not being presented as containers of sexual pollution and moral pathology, they are reduced to signifiers of abjection and unspeakable impoverishment. In discourse on AIDS from a global perspective, for example, women are often framed as one-dimensional victims who are located in far-away, pitiful developing countries.

While it is certainly important not to caricature women as abject and unspeakable, the irony of this comment is that most HIV-positive women are in fact located in far-away, pitiful developing countries, or at least in developing countries. Four out of five HIV-positive women in the world live in Africa (Lawson, 1999), yet the vast majority of literature is Western and presumes a Western audience and a Western subject. Conversely, constructions of the category 'African AIDS' have led to implications that the AIDS found in Africa is foreign and related to a mysterious set of 'African' processes. It has, for example, become interwoven with tropical and distant associations (Seidel, 1993), as well as associations of bestiality and aberrant sexuality (Patton, 1993). This distinguishing of 'African AIDS' is potentially laden with racist assumptions. Patton (1990) suggests that social and medical science are often guilty of 'inventing "African AIDS"' such that much of the resultant work inscribes difference and exoticises Africa rather than attempting to ground analysis in a realistic understanding of

Africa's needs. To view this literature as more culturally sensitive simply because it more often takes Africa as its object of study, then, is not always unproblematic. Patton (1990: 77) warns as follows:

> Debates about ethics in particular occur in a middle ground between two cultures, but the 'second voice' (the 'African perspective') is carried by Western ethicists and researchers who speak of an 'African culture' based largely in their fantasies. In this middle ground of pretended cultural sensitivity, virtually the only audible speech is that which occurs within, or is translated into, the conceptual categories of the modern Western *episteme*.

Whether an African subject or an African culture exists outside of anyone's fantasies, however, is highly debatable. Further, the devastation of AIDS on the continent may be fantastical, but it is also real. Encountering the African context in the era of the Western episteme, then, perhaps inevitably involves balancing a tightrope of negotiation between valuing the differences an African setting brings and resisting patronising assumptions that Africa is so unique and different as to be incomprehensible to outsiders. Comments such as Patton's, therefore, risk taking on a level of paranoia that leads to paralysis rather than to culturally sensitive understanding. The challenge is to understand African AIDS as both typical and unique and to hold a strong African voice and a strong general stance.

In order to avoid repeating these splits, I understand the task of providing context as inherently contradictory and inevitably incomplete. It is often considered important to contextualise studies conducted outside the West. The assumption is that the correct descriptions will render the (unknown) objects of study known and graspable. But perhaps all that can be expected is that contextualisation ignites both expected and unexpected ruminations and images. The imperative to provide context often implicitly holds assumptions about difference – about the need to explain the exotic and unknown. If participants were British, for example, it would be conceivably possible to provide very little context and assume some shared sense of reality between reader (whether British or not) and research participants. Providing context is thus potentially a task that requires explaining where difference and exoticism lies, and thereby in turn holds potential for homogenising and inscribing difference.

The women I interviewed, despite their cultural, economic and environmental landscape, are in many ways not different or strange: they conduct relationships; they have similar hopes and fears to those of other women; they are mothers just like other mothers. At the same time, however, they live within a particular context that is not necessarily familiar to those living outside South Africa (or, indeed, to some living within South Africa), and which informs their subjectivities and their material existence. They are simultaneously familiar and strange, and need to be contextualised as both strange and familiar.

Given the paradoxical nature of the task of 'mapping context', I will avoid abstract depictions of this particular context. Instead, I will describe the research context and then introduce four women who participated in the study, and whose stories vividly illustrate aspects of the social environment. A description of the milieu in which they live will emerge from (inevitably incomplete) exploration of their personal stories; in this way, it is hoped that context will be portrayed as fluid: as both general and unique, familiar and strange.

THE INTERVIEW SETTING

The women who participated in interviews were black women between the ages of 21 and 38. All had some level of schooling, but only one had received a university education. Sixty per cent were unemployed. About a third of the sample were first time mothers. Two women were interviewed who had been diagnosed as HIV-positive before falling pregnant. It is possible that other women were diagnosed before pregnancy, but were unwilling to admit this. About two-thirds were in a relationship of some sort with the fathers of their babies, although many feared that the relationship was breaking down and few actually lived with their partners. Of those who were not in a relationship with their babies' fathers, more than half reported that their partners had left them after they had disclosed their HIV status. Many had also not told family members and had spoken to few people outside the clinic context.

The women interviewed were not a statistical minority. HIV statistics, such as the prevalence of infection among pregnant women, confront one with the sheer enormity of the pandemic, as well as its relevance for Africa and for women. For example, of the 33 million people infected worldwide, 22 million (or 67 per cent) live in sub-Saharan Africa, which is inhabited by just over 10 per cent of the world's population (UNAIDS, 2008). This is not, however, necessarily comforting to those living outside the region. UNAIDS (2004) indicates that HIV infection is on the rise globally, particularly among women in every region of the world. For example, heterosexual infection in Western Europe more than doubled between 1997 and 2002, and HIV has been identified as the fastest-growing health problem in the United Kingdom.

South Africa has the highest number of HIV-infected people in the world at 5.7 million. South African women under 30 are particularly vulnerable (UNAIDS, 2008), i.e. women of childbearing age. HIV may produce marginalised identities, but statistics make clear that HIV-infected South African mothers are in the mainstream and not the margins.

Most women attending clinics were not first-language English speakers. An interpreter could have been used in interviews, but given the confidential and personal nature of interview discussion, it seemed that this would be too intrusive and threatening of confidentiality. Also, interpreter errors are common (Swartz, 1998) and may be ideological in nature (Gentzler, 1993; Venuti, 1992). The use of an interpreter might therefore have compromised the conversations, since HIV is discourse laden in South Africa. This meant that women who did not feel comfortable communicating in English were implicitly excluded from the study. However, South Africa is a multilingual society and many women felt comfortable conversing in English, preferring this to having an interpreter present. It also seemed that many women wanted to participate in interviews and wanted to make themselves understood. In some interviews with women whose English proficiency was relatively poor, they were nonetheless adept at communicating what was important to them: while their language use may not have been sophisticated, their ability to communicate their experience was.

Women were invited to conduct one or more interviews with me, with the flexibility to choose what they felt comfortable revealing. Two-thirds of the sample decided to conduct more than one interview. Second and subsequent interviews held the advantage of deepening interview data, as well as allowing comparison for verification of data and analysis, and for opportunities to examine shifts, continuities and contradictions (Hollway & Jefferson, 2000).

THE CLINIC CONTEXT

The hospital where the research was based is a general hospital, but is known in Johannesburg as a treatment centre for HIV-positive mothers. It is a state hospital and, in contrast to expensive private hospitals, is crowded and understaffed, with limited facilities. All HIV-positive women at this hospital were offered Nevirapine for prevention of mother-to-child transmission in order to reduce the possibility that mothers would transmit the virus to their children. The mechanisms of mother-to-child transmission are very specific. There are three points at which a mother may infect her child: in utero (where there is a 7 per cent chance of infection), during labour or delivery (23 per cent) or through breastfeeding (8 per cent). The cumulative probability of a woman transmitting the virus is estimated at 31 per cent (Department of Health, 2002). Infection rates are reduced if the mother does not breastfeed. Nevirapine is an inexpensive antiretroviral drug that requires minimum dosage to be effective. A single dose of Nevirapine given to the mother before delivery and to the child after birth reduces the probability of mother-to-child transmission by more than half, from

31 per cent to 13 per cent (Department of Health, 2002). Before 2001 this cost only US$4 or, as one comparison acerbically notes, the price of an espresso and croissant.[1] Since then, the cost has dropped dramatically. Transmission modes and rates indicate that the majority of children born to HIV-positive mothers are not infected (59 per cent) and that it is not possible for a mother to transmit HIV to her child through normal maternal care. Expectations of maternal infectiousness, therefore, far exceed reality. Few women interviewed received antiretroviral treatment, which was unavailable at the time of the interviews (2003–04). Although the South African government has agreed to provide antiretroviral treatment for all, the rollout of such treatment has been dogged by controversy and has been perceived to be too slow. In 2004 few South Africans infected with HIV had actually been given treatment (TAC, 2004), while in 2008, it was estimated that 524,000 people requiring treatment were not receiving it (TAC, 2008). Unofficially, overextended hospitals seldom provide symptomatic treatment for opportunistic infections, particularly if it is clear that a patient is in the latter stages of the disease, such that people being refused treatment from hospitals has become a frequent occurrence.

The hospital offers three HIV clinics per week. The antenatal clinic for pregnant women monitors their pregnancy, offers psychoeducational counselling and provides the dose of Nevirapine required before labour. The dose required for the baby after birth is administered in the wards. The postnatal clinic monitors babies for the first year after birth. At the time of the study (2003–04), some women were on a trial designed to establish the efficacy of testing babies' HIV status at four months. Those who were not on the trial had their babies tested when they were one year old. I attended clinics each week and recruited from both. An additional postnatal clinic was run for sick babies. I was advised by the staff not to attend this clinic, because it was predominantly attended by mothers who had refused to test or, when mothers were sick or dead, family members who did not necessarily know the mother's status: my presence would have

1   <http://www.globalstrategies.org>.

risked revealing mothers' and babies' status. The clinic most visibly affected by HIV was thus the most invisible and secretive.

General antenatal clinics were run every day. The waiting room was usually crowded. On the HIV clinic day, however, the waiting area was deserted and the clinic looked closed. Patients waited in a small side room. The door was always kept firmly closed. One had to knock and wait to be admitted. The group began early in the morning with a prayer. While women waited to be seen by a doctor, counsellors addressed various topics, including condom use (the demonstration of which prompted mirth or condescension), facts about the transmission of HIV, guidelines for healthy living and the use of Nevirapine. Most women I interviewed enjoyed these clinics, because they could exchange their stories and observe the psychological and physical strength of others. Most women were at least six months pregnant, partly because clinic visits were more frequent in later pregnancy and partly because many women are diagnosed late in pregnancy (either because they are referred late from local clinics who have not offered tests or because they only went to clinics late in their pregnancies). Five hours later, the group ended with sandwiches and coffee before everybody went home. I interviewed in a private room afterwards (or at other times mutually arranged), since women worried that they would miss seeing a doctor, and if the doctor had already been seen, did not want to miss being in the group.

The postnatal clinic took place in a large ward with beds in the waiting area (for babies to be changed on) and a smaller, cordoned-off consultation area. Unlike the antenatal clinic, the door to the ward was open. In this different setting there was less sense of coherence in the group of those who attended. Women spoke to one another while they waited or listened to counsellors, but they came and left at different times, as well as intermittently fetching their hospital files or fetching formula for their babies, which the hospital provided. Treatment was clearly for their babies, and not themselves: babies were weighed, examined and sometimes tested, but mothers needing medical attention were referred to another hospital. Babies often required attention, and several babies were usually crying at any one time. Participation and involvement in the antenatal group were high; in the postnatal group some women sat centrally to talk to one another, while others sat on the periphery and removed themselves from interaction. Mothers with sick babies were usually on the periphery and often hid their babies under blankets, even in the height of summer, as if ashamed of having them seen. At this clinic, I interviewed throughout the day.

Clinics were predominantly attended by black women. In the six months in which I visited clinics, one white woman attended one session. One of the counsellors told me that there were so few coloured women at the HIV clinic because, she thought, stigma was stronger in this community: coloured women diagnosed as HIV-positive were generally apprehensive to attend the group for fear of being recognised and labelled.[2] Few staff members were white. Because I am white, patients presumed I was not a patient and was part of the medical team. 'Race' remains a visible issue in South Africa, and I had expected racial difference to be an important dynamic in interviews. On my first day in the antenatal clinic, I was greeted with suspicion by the mothers, partly because they were mistrustful of what I might think of them. In discussion, scepticism was voiced regarding whether I, as a white woman, would be able to understand their experiences. They were more concerned, however, about whether I would respect their confidentiality, their immediate assumption being that I would divulge their identities to the press. Some were also suspicious about the participation fee I offered: one woman said that her story was not for sale. We discussed these concerns, and the women concluded that they would need time to think about whether they would like to participate or not.

The next time I attended the clinic, however, the atmosphere was very different, and throughout the research period more women wanted to participate in the research than time allowed. The counsellors were at least partly responsible for this. Overstretched and underpaid, working without

2 This category was constructed during the apartheid era in order to indicate people of mixed racial heritage. The term continues to be used.

supervision, they were eager for me to interview the women, since they could not listen to everybody. The women seemed to observe mutual respect between myself and counsellors, and to be more eager to participate as a result. They also spoke to one another, and a number of women decided to participate after a friend had told them about her own interview. The majority of women had few people to talk to, and commented on how difficult it was to find someone discreet and non-judgmental with whom to talk for any significant period of time.

Within this context, issues of racial difference seemed to become less important. Participants often assumed, for example, that I understood aspects of their cultural and racial environment. Other differences, such as my HIV-negative status, my qualifications and my status as non-mother seemed more important, but were infrequently mentioned. Although a few women seemed primarily motivated by the research fee and some by a desire to help others, most of them treated interviews as an opportunity to gain some relief or understanding of themselves, and often verbalised this explicitly.

My HIV status was occasionally commented on in interviews. One woman told me to be sure to use condoms and stay HIV-negative. Another, assuming that white people do not get HIV, asked me why this was the case. When I was in the clinic, however, it seemed that women sometimes tested me. For example, I was requested to share food, cups or lipstick while frequently being told in interviews about those who refused to share such things because they were afraid of HIV-positive people. Few people asked whether I was a mother or not. Interestingly, this became more prevalent towards the end of the research for some women who had conducted several interviews with me. One, for example, felt that I should not delay motherhood, because 'it's nice', while another said I probably wanted to be a mother, but that it would be better for me to remain childless. The fact that I am a clinical psychologist was perhaps most commented on: participants often asked me for answers and a number of women described wanting to study further and being unable to afford to do so. One woman said she had wanted to be a social worker or psychologist like me, but had no money to do so. This was a comment on her lack of education compared to mine, but also on my affluence compared to hers. It was thus the difference of socioeconomic status that was most visible in interviews (but, of course, not in all interviews). For example, a number of women asked me to help them find employment. A few who were relatively economically secure took pains to describe how they had grown up in poverty. In a number of interviews, women described their poverty in ways that suggested that they thought I would be least able to understand this aspect of their lives. My whiteness, socioeconomic status and presence in the hospital frequently led to assumptions that I was a doctor, and the expectation that I would be helpful seemed to mitigate markers of difference. Further, many women made comments implying that they felt I could identify with them because I was a woman: it seemed that, in talking about HIV-positive motherhood, gender was more important than race.

The research setting, both within clinics and interviews, was a very specific context strongly influenced by the medical institution in which it was positioned, as well as, of course, by the ever-presence of HIV and motherhood that defined its very existence. It was a complex environment that allowed sharing and connection, but was also marked by remembrance and alienation – the clinic and the interviews reminded women of their HIV-positive status and were defined not only by the inclusion of acceptance, but by the alienation that separated HIV-positive mothers (who belonged in these clinics) from everybody else (who did not). It was an environment that allowed or disallowed different things for different women and to which a range of experiences, backgrounds and emotions were brought. While most women were black, they came from a variety of different places and spoke a number of different languages. While they were generally poor, the women's socioeconomic environment varied. Some held culture and tradition to be important, while others considered themselves 'modern' urban women. Some women had conservative approaches to gender relations, while others felt themselves to be more liberal. Some lived their lives independently; others held deep and valued connections to their extended family, religion or other institutions. At the same time, the social environment held similarities for many women.

The remainder of this chapter focuses on introducing four of the women I interviewed. The different aspects of their stories are gathered together here to introduce the complexity of their situations. Many of the themes that arise in these stories are echoed across the narratives of the other women. These particular cases, which are abundant with disparities, serve to offer a sense of the wide-ranging experiences of HIV-positive mothers in the broader context of their lives, and to foreground for the reader, before some of the theoretical issues of motherhood are introduced, the realities of everyday life and the centrality of the women's stories to this book.

HLENGIWE

Hlengiwe, eight months pregnant with her first child, was diagnosed HIV-positive two months previously. She is employed and, like many women with or without partners, lives with family members, in this case her cousins. On the day of the interview, she was wearing a short, bright sundress and was vibrantly attractive. She has been together with her boyfriend for the past three years, and has told him, but no-one else, of her status. She is not sure who brought HIV into the relationship. She describes her boyfriend as supportive, but she worries that he has continued drinking excessively. She worries about his health, but also suspects he is drinking in order to avoid talking to her: 'to the person always drunk … maybe you cannot hear those things maybe she wants to say to you and all. I don't know.' When she told him of her status, she shared the concern of many women that he would leave her:

> Mm, in terms of the HIV, I think he's done better compared to other men, because if you tell them that you are HIV, they run away, but he didn't. … But I said to him, 'But the way you are acting, eh, for me, I do understand that it's difficult, but you make me suspicious; I cannot rest. But I have to be prepared; I know I'm stronger. I have to

be prepared and you know what, you'll deal with this alone; maybe you'll deal with it alone.' Then he said, 'no, I'll never do that.' But you never know.

She remains unconvinced that he will not leave her.

Like many others, Hlengiwe was brought up by grandparents – in this case both her paternal and maternal grandmothers. Her father has a wife and three children, including herself. She feels that her mother may blame her for the fact that she is not together with Hlengiwe's father, and imagines her mother thinking, 'my life is a mess because of [Hlengiwe]; if I was not pregnant [with Hlengiwe], maybe I would still be going out with her father'. Hlengiwe understands that her mother could not support her financially, but feels rejected by her:

> I understand that she's not working and there's nothing maybe she can do for me, but as a mother, even if, according to me, you are not working doesn't mean you have to shut your whole world. The love it's there and the love makes another person grow. Somewhere, somehow I resent my mother; I don't like her so much. *Ja*.

Her mother has not seen her since she became pregnant. She feels isolated from her family, alone both emotionally and financially and forced to rely on her boyfriend. For example, she explained that she started a tertiary qualification after she finished school, but did not complete the first year, because she was unable to pay her fees.

> So [my family] know nothing about me, they just brought me, in our culture when you are 21, you have to see for yourself, but how can you see for yourself if you are not working, if you do not have an education? … How can I work a professional job, yet I'm not educated? You see, Carol, such things?

It should be noted that it is not necessarily culturally the case that adults are left to fend for themselves; it was expected that family members would look after one another, and more specifically that participants had obligations to financially support siblings and parents. Hlengiwe, however, felt she could rely on nobody.

This, combined with the powerful social stigma associated with HIV, prevented her from disclosing her status to others:

> Yes, maybe they can blame you: '*Ja*, you, because you live alone, that's why you are like this today. You hang around men.' All these things because they don't understand; they live where they live; their life, it's fine, but if you start disclosing this information – because they take HIV/AIDS, I'm sorry to say that, a bitch or what, you know, such things, not knowing how did you get that, but because you are HIV, it means you have been sleeping around and sleeping, sleeping around.

Hlengiwe's fears of being labelled echo statements made throughout interviews, but are specifically framed by her own story, particularly her independence and isolation from her family: 'because you live alone.'

Just before Hlengiwe participated in the interview, she discovered at the clinic that the Nevirapine treatment offered does not guarantee that her baby will be negative. She was shocked, as she had presumed her baby would automatically be safe. She had also not been aware that she would have to wait a considerable period of time before she knew her baby's test result. Having very recently discovered that she was HIV-positive, the shock of facing this uncertainty regarding her baby was devastating news. She became tearful in the interview when contemplating the implications. This was a primary concern for all women interviewed, and the pervasiveness of this uncertainty was present in the postnatal clinic, where some women were still waiting for their babies' results.

Because Hlengiwe knew that HIV can be transmitted through breast milk, she had decided not to breastfeed (as had all the women I interviewed).

The probability of transmitting the virus while breastfeeding depends upon a number of factors and is reduced if exclusive breastfeeding is undertaken (Coutsoudis, 2005). There is some debate regarding whether women should be discouraged from breastfeeding or not. Exclusive breastfeeding is difficult to adhere to in economically challenged environments (Thairu et al., 2005), but it has been argued that the advantages of breast milk for overall mortality outweigh the risks of possible infection (Bland et al., 2002; Coutsoudis et al., 2003). This dilemma is complicated by beliefs and practices. For example, Kruger and Gericke (2003) found that all their research participants believed that breast is best (thereby problematising the use of formula feed), but none believed in exclusive breastfeeding. Hlengiwe, like most of the women interviewed, was not aware of this debate, but had definitively decided not to breastfeed. She was worried, however, that this would be interpreted as a sign that she is a bad mother or as an indication that she is HIV-positive. It is culturally expected that an African woman should breastfeed openly in public, and this is understood as the quintessential sign of being a good mother. For many women, this complicated their construction of themselves as 'good mothers'. They were also criticised by family members for being bad mothers. The cultural breast defines the mother; a woman who chooses not to breastfeed is choosing to reject her culture. Even for women who resisted cultural discourses, the cultural imperative to breastfeed had to be addressed. One woman, for example, said she wasn't affected by not breastfeeding, because she had always felt that black women who breastfeed in public do not respect their bodies. Her way of justifying her decision to me could not be done without reference to culture. The cultural implications of choosing not to breastfeed are further complicated by the social assumptions that women who do not breastfeed are HIV-positive. Hlengiwe was scared that her secret would be exposed by her choice not to breastfeed, but felt that she had no other choice. In terms of the cultural definition of motherhood, many felt personally bereft of feeling like mothers.

Hlengiwe planned to conduct another interview with me, but cancelled at the last minute because she wanted another woman, who was contemplating adoption, to do an interview instead. She did not want me to contact her for fear of arousing suspicion. I did not see her in the postnatal clinic and she did not contact me. Like all the stories in this study, my telling of it is incomplete.

PUMLA

Pumla, unemployed, conducted an interview with me when she was eight months pregnant and again when her son was three months old, before she knew his status. Her appearance was neat and her dress demure. She did not see herself as a 'modern woman', as did Hlengiwe. Pumla was diagnosed HIV-positive when she was three months pregnant. At the time, she was living with her boyfriend of ten years, the only person with whom she had had a sexual relationship. This relationship was stable, but violent; she described how he was hypervigilant of her actions and showed me a scar on her face where he had hit her with a gun. She was not the only woman to describe domestic violence: South Africa has one of the highest domestic and sexual violence rates in the world. Pumla had been concerned that her boyfriend had other sexual partners and, before being diagnosed, had thought about asking him to use a condom. However, she was too scared to do so. Strebel (1997) suggests that South African women are caught in a paradox in which they are expected to take responsibility for safe sex, but are often powerless to do so. The 'good' woman should avoid becoming HIV-positive by maintaining self-control, self-discipline and responsibility (Sacks, 1996). In everyday negotiations, however, expecting women to take responsibility for their sexuality ignores the asymmetry of heterosexual relationships (Kippax et al., 1990). This has particular resonance in Africa, where women have little access to sexual negotiating power (Lawson, 1999). A woman who requests condom use, for example, is likely to be accused of being HIV infected or promiscuous, or of accusing her partner of infidelity (Santow, 1995), the consequences of which can be violent and can lead to economic hardship (Strebel, 1992). This is precisely what

Pumla was scared of. Urging South African women to ask their men to use condoms ignores male suspicion of condoms (Maharaj, 2001), as well as the interaction between male power and discourses of love for women, where women may accept what men want because they love them (Hoosen & Collins, 2004). Further, AIDS campaigns often reinforce the sanctity of faithful heterosexual relationships (Seidel, 1990) without acknowledging double standards in which male promiscuity is acceptable or situations in which multiple sexual partners may signify masculinity (Walker, Reid & Cornell, 2004). In circumstances such as these, a woman's faithfulness, such as Pumla's, to her partner therefore often fails to protect her from HIV infection (Lawson, 1999).

When Pumla told her boyfriend that she was positive, he 'chased' her away, 'and he said to me, "if you call me and accuse me of that, you're wasting your time. You can see me that I'm happy, I'm healthy, I'm okay"'. He accused her of becoming infected through 'sleeping around' and denied any possibility that he may be infected. He had seen the baby once since he was born, but denies paternity.

Left with nowhere to live, Pumla approached her mother and disclosed her status. At first her mother was supportive, but, when her baby was a few days old, told her to leave and not come back: 'I'm finished with your child.' Pumla thinks that her mother assumed that she and her baby would become sick immediately and did not want the scandal associated with an AIDS-related death, that her mother blamed Pumla for becoming infected, and that 'it's my fault, because I didn't listen to her'. When I asked what her relationship with her family had been like before her diagnosis, she said that she was 'very, very close' to her mother:

> You see, I was working and I didn't have a baby, you know. It was
> my mother, and my mother she is a pensioner, and my brother and
> my sister, né, who stay with my mother. So my mother, she loved me
> very, very, very much, because each and everything that I do, when
> I buy groceries, I buy groceries for my mother, because I'm working

and I have money. Every time when I bought something, it's for my mother, because I know that my brother he's drinking, you see all these things, and my sister can't help my mother. Everything was very, very good; me and my mother got on well.

This illustrates the cultural importance of supporting one's family, a value shared by most participants, whether they lived with family or not. For Pumla, however, this support was not reciprocated and she was forced to live on her own. This was particularly hurtful for her, given the culturally accepted practice that a woman lives with her mother after a baby is born so her mother can help with the first stages of childrearing and protect her in the maternal home. Even women who lived with their partners were expected to go to their mothers' homes for a period post-partum. In reality, however, few women were able to do this, either because their mothers lived far away, were old or had died; because they had difficult relationships with their mothers; or because they were stigmatised and rejected because of their HIV status, as in Pumla's case.

Although some women were supported after disclosing their HIV status, all the women interviewed experienced some stigma. This was sometimes a direct result of disclosing their status, but was sometimes indirect. Numerous examples were cited of women overhearing or participating in conversations about HIV with people who did not know that they were positive and being hurt by the prejudiced comments people made. Pumla describes a typical example in which this prejudice is combined with assumptions about motherhood:

Whenever these people they talk about HIV and AIDS [and] they think people [are] with HIV, people like to talk very, very, very bad things about HIV people. Sometimes they say, 'oh, I don't like these people. If maybe somebody can come into my house and say they're HIV-positive, I can say, 'no you must go'. Then I said to this person, 'if I can tell you that I'm HIV-positive, what are you going to do?' He said to me, 'no, I can see that you are clean. You've got a small child. If you were having HIV, people with HIV, the children they die, so I can see your baby is growing normally and you're healthy too.'

The assumption here is that mothers who are 'clean' cannot be 'bad' or HIV-positive. Pumla describes becoming increasingly expectant of being rejected on the basis of her HIV status. She felt stigmatised against, even by the hospital. She described telling an HIV-positive friend about a recent conversation with her doctor, who warned her not to touch her baby, even though medical opinion is virtually unanimous that you cannot give some HIV by touching them:

I said, '[the doctor said,] do you know that if you, you are positive, you mustn't kiss your child, mustn't sleep with your child with you'. She said to me, '*hau!*' Then I said, 'the doctor said even if you give them food, you mustn't taste anything'.

HIV transmission was a primary concern for many. The women I interviewed, including Pumla, were well informed about modes of transmission. Many kept newspaper clippings and voraciously watched television programmes in order to keep themselves informed. They understood that HIV can be transmitted during pregnancy and labour or through breast milk. Similarly, they knew that normal physical contact is perfectly safe. Many described the social prejudice that physical contact could be contagious. Pumla knew that kissing her baby or sharing food did not put her baby at risk, but doubted her knowledge in the face of medical opinion. It is unclear whether a doctor actually said this; and it is unlikely that the doctors at the treating hospital would have expressed this stigmatised view, but the doctor she described was at a local clinic. In a sense, it is immaterial whether this was actually said or not. For Pumla, this idea simultaneously expressed her anger at being stigmatised and her fears of infecting her baby.

She also described attempting to gain support from her church. Christianity was important to her, as to many participants, and so she spoke to the priest's wife. Having experienced prejudice, she framed it carefully: 'I didn't say I'm positive to the lady. I say they think that I might be positive.' In her view, her wariness was justified; she thought that the priest's wife had betrayed her confidence:

> Sunday, when I go to church, the priest was busy preaching about people who don't respect their mothers and some of them they are HIV-positive; yes, you see, if you're HIV-positive, you've done bad things to your body. God shows that you, you see [inaudible]. So this lady told him and that's why he was preaching like that.

In a context where HIV awareness is visible on television, in newspapers, in schools and on billboards, the ostracism that circulates in the face of HIV is striking. Pumla described stigma in her social environment and also described how she cherished a television advertisement showing a white man who had lived with HIV for 19 years. Pumla felt particularly trapped by her status and described feeling self-anger and self-hatred for becoming HIV-positive. The contradiction that it wasn't her fault, but that she was to blame, a contradiction shared by other women, was one that she was unable to resolve, and one that was echoed in the social environment.

LELETI

Leleti was diagnosed HIV-positive just before giving birth to her son. She attended a local clinic where no routine testing took place, but 'luckily', she says, her baby was in the breech position and she was sent to the clinic where my interview with her took place. She was unemployed and lived with her mother, with whom she had a close relationship. Her son, seven months old, was HIV-negative. Leleti conducted two interviews with me, deciding to participate on the suggestion of counsellors, because she was tearful and in mourning. Her boyfriend had recently died, probably of an AIDS-related illness. She had told him of her diagnosis when she was pregnant and he had been accepting and loving, had gone for a test himself, but had been too scared to return for the results. He had later become rapidly sicker within a week; his death had been unexpected. Since his death, his family had completely ostracised her and had left her financially destitute. She feels they may blame her for his death: 'I don't know, maybe they think I'm, I killed him, I don't know. I don't know what they are thinking, but it seems like, like it's that.'

Leleti has not disclosed her status to anyone else. She is particularly reluctant to tell her mother, whom she feels is too old and fragile and may not cope with another loss: 'I don't know how it's going to be [if I tell her,] because ... she had her heart broken with my boyfriend.' The implication in the interview was that Leleti knew about broken hearts. Leleti's brother died many years previously from an unexplained illness and this loss was brought back to her when her boyfriend died: 'it's a double loss now, you know.' She had also previously lost her first infant son, who had been sick since birth and would not get better. She did not explicitly say that this loss may have been AIDS related, almost as though it were too painful to voice, but she had clearly wondered whether it was. She thanked God, for example, for allowing her to save this new baby, and also said that if she had known her status with her first baby, 'maybe he was going to be alive by now'.

Leleti's HIV diagnosis, therefore, was not isolated in her body and mind, but was intimately connected with the AIDS-related deaths of others. In South Africa, where heterosexual contact is the primary mode of transmission and infection rates are high, HIV is not an exception and does not exist in the margins of society. Leleti's contemplation of her own death took place in the context of having seen others die. This was common: almost everybody spoke about the experience of watching somebody – either a loved one or a neighbour – becoming sick and dying. Kuli and Nonyameko, for example, had lost babies to AIDS. Palesa's brother had full-blown AIDS, but they were both too scared to tell one another their shared status. Amara bumped into her sister at an HIV clinic. Both pretended that they were not at an HIV clinic and that nothing had been disclosed. Neither spoke about it again. Joyce nursed her mother through an AIDS-related death a few years before being diagnosed herself. AIDS-related death is therefore powerfully present in the social domain, in everyday conversation and in observation. Its presence is, however, both explicitly known and explicitly hidden. People proudly wear HIV-positive t-shirts, but there are many funerals in which the cause of death is not stated. A counsellor joked to me about a funeral poster in the hospital that, like many others, was so silent about cause of death that it told everybody what was actually going on, and everybody understood.

Leleti felt herself caught in this social milieu of disclosure and silence. She was scared to disclose her status, but at the same time wanted to tell people about her status and about 'the disease and all that ... I feel like I can talk to people. Maybe I can be healed somewhere, somehow, you know, at least to live long.' This desire was linked to her experience of encountering other HIV-positive women at the clinic. This often allowed comparisons that helped to disperse feelings of badness. Some women saw that others were healthy and felt they could be so too. Some saw others as moral women, some saw courage and others saw good mothers. Leleti, who was deeply religious, said that 'I was not the only one who said that maybe God doesn't love me, or all that. It's just happened, you know, so I must accept it that I should live long or, you know.'

Leleti found strength in being known and seen as HIV-positive at the clinic. Her fear of being known and seen more publicly, however, was not only for herself. She was scared, like many women, that people would treat her son differently, even though he was HIV-negative. She felt that she could not ask her mother to care for her son after her death, because her mother was too old, or her sisters, because they had their own families. She worried about anybody else caring for her child, because of the implications if her status were known:

Because in our culture, sometimes they say if people are thinking about the baby, if they want the baby dead, they don't want the baby, sometimes the baby can get sick and all that, you know those, uh, that stuff. But it's true sometimes, you know. So I just want, I don't want them near my baby.

Her fear, related to the cultural belief that malicious thoughts bring malicious consequences, was about her son being harmed because prejudice directed towards herself as HIV-positive would be carried over to him. She was thus caught between hoping that going public would heal her and fearing that the reactions of others would have harmful consequences for her baby. Leleti had experienced both loss and rejection – with very practical financial consequences – as a result of AIDS.

NOMBEKO

Nombeko is an unemployed single mother who was diagnosed HIV-positive when she was five months pregnant. Her HIV-negative son was a year old when I met her. She lives in Johannesburg with her mother, although her hometown is in a rural area. She has strong roots in both traditional and urban identities. She considers herself a modern woman aspiring to Western ideals, but is also respectful and observant of traditional values and practices. Her father died when she was a child and her older brother died when she was a young adult. She has no other siblings, and speaks of herself as an only child. Her mother has an underpaid job, and Nombeko has little money. She worries that she is supposed to eat properly in order to maintain her health, but cannot afford to do so. Her mother knows she is HIV-positive, but no other family members know. She has told friends in Johannesburg, but feels unable to disclose in her hometown. Her HIV-positive status is an important part of her identity; she is eager to talk to people about HIV and, like many women interviewed, has strong desires to become an HIV counsellor. She and a friend initiated a group offering HIV education, and they were securing funding to get it started.

Nombeko is not sure how she contracted HIV. She says she only slept with the father of her baby on one occasion; she wondered at times whether she contracted HIV from him. At our first interview, he had not yet seen his son, refusing to have anything to do with him or Nombeko. Before our fourth interview, she was diagnosed with syphilis and, realising that she had previously had symptoms, wondered whether she had been HIV-positive for five years. The father of her baby comes from her hometown. In our first interview, she said he had slept with at least four other women that she knows of. Her guess was that he refused to wear a condom (as he had refused with her) and that these women may also have become infected.

She is a member of the Zionist Christian Church (ZCC), a popular evangelical church with links to African traditional practices and with a strong presence in the community. Many women I interviewed had roots in both Christianity and traditional belief systems. The ZCC brings these traditions together; e.g. the priest is also the healer. Traditional beliefs about health and illness are often believed to be a message or punishment from the ancestors or connected to bewitchment. Nombeko explained the many beliefs about HIV that were strong in her hometown. South Africans have a wide array of easily available AIDS myths to construct AIDS as somebody else's problem. The common belief that only black people get AIDS (Robins, 2004) makes other population groups feel safer. Similarly, the belief that only promiscuous women contract AIDS makes promiscuous men feel safer (Maharaj, 2001). AIDS interacts with discourses of race, culture and gender to construct systems of safety and morality. Robins (2004: 654) lists some of the many myths in common circulation:

> The blaming of AIDS on witchcraft, as well as a variety of AIDS conspiracies: 'whites' who want to contain black population growth; 'white doctors' who inject patients with AIDS when they go for tests; the CIA and pharmaceutical companies who want to create markets for drugs in Africa; the use of Africans as guinea pigs for scientific

experiments with AIDS drugs; beliefs that sex with virgins, including infants, can cure AIDS; as well as beliefs that anti-retrovirals are dangerously toxic and that the lubricant in condoms is a source of HIV infection.

Nombeko was concerned about the array of myths on offer. She explained, for example, that

> in our culture, they said if I can sleep with a man who's wife is dead, I'll get sick. They are taking HIV as like, just like that, you know, like it's not a killing disease; they will just cure it and then go away.

Nombeko is referring to a common belief that having sex with a widowed man during his period of mourning angers the ancestors, who then make the woman sick. If she can appease the ancestors, she will be cured. At the same time, there are strong beliefs that whatever happens is God's will, and only God can cure people. Nombeko described people who would come to her church to be cured, but at the same time, these church members believed that it was impossible for them, as God's children, to contract HIV. According to these traditions, illness is taken to a church or traditional healer. Many consult medical practitioners as well, despite their contradictory frameworks and practices (Lund & Swartz, 1998). Nombeko believed in the power of the church and of traditional healers, but, echoing other women, was adamant that they could not help with HIV and should not be consulted. She angrily described people who say that HIV is 'witchcraft' and that somebody 'didn't like her; maybe that's why they did this to her. You know, they are all in very big denial stage at home.' For her, traditional medicine and Christian beliefs work, but not for HIV:

> You know there, like, they said, you can hear how they say there's someone who can cure you, whatever. I said, 'you know, this disease, it's like an English disease. It's like it can't cure by the sangomas [traditional

healers], whatever.' [She then explains that people mistake HIV for bewitchment or failure to adhere to cultural practice.] They are taking it, they want to convert it to tradition, to those things. But it can't. It just isn't. It's HIV. It's HIV, it's a virus, it's in your blood, you know.

Nombeko, at least in the hospital context, separates HIV from her experience with other diseases. Only medical doctors can help, because it is an 'English disease' that is not amenable to African cures. Surprisingly few women discussed traditional practices at length during interviews, no doubt partly because of the influence of the hospital context and my association with it. Nombeko positions herself as both traditional and anti-traditional; HIV is, however, firmly situated in the medical realm.

I met with Nombeko four times over a period of four months. She is a well-dressed and well-groomed woman who pays close attention to her appearance. She is very thin, with abrasions on her skin. She said several times that friends or acquaintances commented on how fat and healthy she appeared, which further highlighted how thin she actually was.

In her first interview, Nombeko spoke at length about her horror at the spread of HIV/AIDS. This was related to her feelings of guilt that she may be responsible for infecting women who had slept with her baby's father – because she had not told them about her own status, rather than because she feared she had indirectly spread HIV to them. Respondents seldom verbalised thinking of the infection of other women through their partners; Nombeko was atypical in voicing such concerns.

The second interview started with my asking her how things were going with her. She replied:

Oh, it's like now, I think I can deal with it now. *Ja.* But some days I can, some days I cannot; but these days that I can say 'thank God I can', it's like when I'm talking to somebody, like you, like that lady I'm working with, it's better. But I can spend the whole day not talking to anybody; it's like eating me inside.

Nombeko's opening assertion 'I think I can deal with it now' seems strong, but it immediately wavers into 'it's eating me inside'. The struggle between being 'brave' (a word she frequently used) and not coping characterised the narrative structure of her interviews, connected here to her interactions with other people. She spoke about the support group she was starting – 'You know, it means a lot to me, it's like I'm doing something ... I even feel like a[n HIV-]negative person' – but soon switched to telling stories about watching people dying. Sickness and death were more present in this interview than the first, as were statements about the need for courage and acceptance. I came away from the interview feeling that her statements of hope were haunted by dead and dying bodies. Discussions of motherhood felt as though they were somehow separate, but couldn't be separated fully. For example, she imagined telling friends that she was HIV-positive and not being believed, because her baby was 'healthy, you know, nice and everything, how can I be positive?' – as if HIV and motherhood were mutually exclusive.

Before our third interview, the hospital had contacted Nombeko to request another blood test to confirm her son's negative status. She had not expected another test, and felt that the closure that she had reached regarding her son's status had been reversed: 'It's like it's repeating itself all over again.' She spoke more, however, about her own HIV-positive status than her child's status in the interview, and I wondered whether the sense of regression she described regarding her son's status had underscored the fact that she was HIV-positive. There was more discussion in this interview about sickness and death, often in the context of discussions of broader social systems (such as the church, traditional healing and the hospital). If the central metaphor in the first interview was that of the spread of HIV, the central metaphor here was of a social system trying, and failing, to ignore death. Towards the end of the interview, she said that her mother had found a new boyfriend. Nombeko was terrified that he would infect her mother, but was too scared to discuss this with her, because it transgressed culturally acceptable relations of respect between mothers and daughters. She was worried that if her mother became infected, she would not be able to look after Nombeko when she became sick, or Nombeko's son when Nombeko died.

In the fourth interview, events had intervened again to foreground sickness and death. Nombeko had been diagnosed with syphilis and told that it may become neurological if she did not follow treatment. This provoked anxiety about her body and, in conjunction with the request for a further HIV test for her son, about his body. Discussion of monitoring the body was common among most respondents, and had been present in previous interviews with Nombeko, but was strongly expressed in this interview. The interview occurred before she was due to go back to her rural home, and she was worried about seeing her baby's father and fearful of encountering people dying of AIDS at home, where she felt she could not disclose her own status for fear of rejection. The interview ended on a triumphant note as she told me she had successfully spoken to her mother, asked her not to have sex without a condom and explained her concerns. Her mother was proud of her, as was Nombeko, for having the strength to talk.

Nombeko had wanted a final interview, but could not afford to return to Johannesburg. When we spoke on the telephone, she said she had been reunited with her son's father, at first as a coerced reunion, but then he had become progressively more open and she was optimistic about their relationship. Her son's negative status was confirmed. She had been sick, and said she had lost weight. When we ended our last telephone conversation, she laughingly said that I should not worry, because she would still be alive when I returned to South Africa. I put the telephone down with the sinking feeling that perhaps she would not be.

CONCLUSION

For the four women introduced above, an HIV-positive diagnosis was intertwined with family relationships, gender relations, social and cultural norms and beliefs, and financial hardship, as well as with the practicalities of living with HIV, including the need to live a healthy lifestyle, to forego breastfeeding and to face the uncertainty of their baby's HIV status for at least a period of time. In this telling, context has not been fully or accurately described, but has been partially described through the lens of particular women, their telling of what has been important and my retelling of their setting. Inevitably in the telling, certain aspects run the risk of becoming objective realities when they are not. These stories only begin to describe events and experiences in a particular time and place, but tell something of the contradictions and challenges encountered.

Each woman tells a story that is simultaneously intimately personal and indelibly social. In each story, AIDS discourse constructs how women are understood by others and by themselves. HIV/AIDS is distinctly a disease that has lent itself to metaphor (Sontag, 1988). Although many illnesses could be considered metaphoric, Sontag (1988) argues that AIDS becomes particularly so because it is linked to sexuality and perversity and because it therefore inscribes itself on the identity of the HIV-positive person. Other diseases share this link, but AIDS dominates the metaphorical market: 'It seems that societies need to have one illness which becomes identified with evil, and attaches blame to its "victims", but it is hard to be obsessed with more than one' (Sontag, 1988: 16). Because of its associated stigma, it has been argued that HIV/AIDS cannot be understood outside the social systems of meaning that inscribe the HIV-positive (and -negative) body. This makes HIV/AIDS an 'epidemic of signification' (Treichler, 1988: 31), implying that it has prompted an epidemic of meanings and also that these meanings fuel and perpetuate the escalation of the epidemic. Treichler (1988) suggests that AIDS discourse proliferates by linking to pre-existing systems of difference, thereby making 'us' feel safe. It has therefore been suggested that investigation into the significations attached to HIV/AIDS is far from an abstract enterprise, since these meanings directly relate to social policy and practice and to the experience of being HIV-positive (Seidel, 1990). Understanding these meanings is central to curbing the epidemic (Strebel, 1997) and to a better understanding of the ways in which these meanings construct HIV-positive subjectivity (Willig, 2000). AIDS discourse is not simply about irrational and politically loaded meaning; it is centrally about the ways in which these social meanings proliferate both themselves and the virus. As matrices of discrimination have strengthened as it became clearer that the virus does not discriminate, so the virus has proliferated as a consequence of this discrimination.

South African HIV-positive motherhood finds itself within a knot of such discrimination. Walker (1990) notes that any South African feminism can only be relevant with a recognition that the majority of women in South Africa are not just women, but face a triple oppression of gender, class and race. South African women who find themselves HIV-positive thus add another type of discrimination, marked as it is by stigma. Considering the powerful fantasies circulating in the social world, the experience of actually becoming HIV-positive brings into experience the laden question of whether one has become these fantasies, as well as the dilemma of finding and defining oneself in relation to HIV and others.

3. The Joys of Motherhood

Stories ... said that Nnu Ego was a wicked woman even in death because, however many people appealed to her to make women fertile, she never did. Poor Nnu Ego, even in death she had no peace! Still, many agreed that she had given all to her children. The joy of being a mother was the joy of giving all to your children, they said ... for what else could a woman want but to have sons who would give her a decent burial? Nnu Ego had it all, yet still did not answer prayers for children.

Buchi Emecheta, *The Joys of Motherhood*

Buchi Emecheta's novel tells of an African woman whose only desire was to be a respected mother, but whose experiences repeatedly confronted her with gaps between social ideals of motherhood and her everyday realities (Christian, 1994). Expecting to be rewarded for having given all to her children, the 'joys' of motherhood turned out to be more complex than she had expected. Diligently implementing the maternal selflessness required of her, she found herself constantly up against hardship and blame, the rewards of motherhood continually deferred and never achieved, except in her bittersweet 'decent burial'. The irony of the title of the novel is that she did achieve the joys of motherhood, but could never entirely live up to social ideals and had never expected the selflessness of giving all to her children to demand such great cost and reap so little reward.

Theoretically, socially and personally, motherhood is often constructed as a function rather than an experience: the subject of motherhood is the child receiving mothering rather than the mother herself. This chapter explores theoretical perspectives on motherhood, drawing on the idea of the 'joys of motherhood' to suggest that motherhood is perhaps the most idealised, exclusive and defining identity associated with womanhood, and that a woman's relation to her reproductive capacities (and therefore her sexuality) is a primary social site for the construction of divisions between 'good' and 'bad' women. Motherhood is expected to be a selfless joy, realised in the joys of the mother's children, rather than a joy owned by herself. While these social ideals may be defining of motherhood, however, it will be suggested that they cannot completely construct mothers: the experience of motherhood from the mother's perspective exists in its own right. This chapter explores dominant constructions of motherhood from a feminist perspective, followed by a psychoanalytic repositioning of motherhood from the mother's point of view. The politics of the category 'South African mother' is then considered.

DECONSTRUCTING MOTHERHOOD

Rich (1977), describing what she calls the institution of motherhood – the ways in which social norms and processes come to form normative images of mothers – highlights 'the floating notion that a woman pregnant is a woman calm in her fulfilment or, simply, a woman waiting' (Rich, 1977: 39). Historical divisions between mother as Madonna and whore (Welldon, 1988) idealise motherhood as a state of purity and, as Rich implies, valorise passivity. This sets up 'ideal mothering [as] endlessly loving, serenely healing, emotionally rewarding'

(O'Barr, Pope & Wyer, 1990: 14). The good mother happily indulges in her labours of love, expecting no rewards, but basking in maternal bliss.

One problem with idealisation, however, is that it sets an impossible standard against which women are expected to measure themselves. Dominant constructions of motherhood naturalise the biological capacity of women to bear children as the pinnacle of female experience (Glenn, 1994) and define the tasks and experience of motherhood in normative ways (Phoenix & Woollett, 1991b). Deconstructing motherhood involves a rejection of unitary truths, highlighting instead that constructions of motherhood participate in, and reproduce, power relations. Feminist interest in the political implications of the category arose most notably in the 1970s, where the importance of motherhood as a site of patriarchal regulation was a key area of feminist theorising. Two often-overlapping issues came to define progressive writing: a concern with the social institution of motherhood and the ways in which it maintains gendered power relations (e.g. Rich, 1977), and a concern with documenting the experiences of mothers, thus reclaiming constructions of motherhood from dominant patriarchal discourses (e.g. Oakley, 1980; Dally, 1982). Feminists continue to argue that constructions of motherhood and issues of reproduction are significant sites for the regulation of women (Marshall & Woollett, 2000). Within these arguments, maternal idealisation prescribes female experience to patriarchal advantage. On the one hand, power relations are maintained, and on the other, motherhood is strictly defined as a female domain: 'By defining mothering as essentially biological, moral, and timeless, the patriarchal state is relieved of the necessity to make material, political, and temporal arrangements to assist it' (O'Barr, Pope & Wyer, 1990: 3).

The suggestion here is that idealisations of motherhood are both active, patriarchally constructing 'good' mothers (actively asserting power over the domain of motherhood), and passive, asserting power by defining the responsibilities of motherhood in naturalised terms.

Theories addressing patriarchal power address the broad consequences of maternal idealisation for the institution of motherhood, but only hint at the implications for maternal experiences. In this regard, it is useful to examine not only what power does, but also what it hides. Because of the pervasiveness of idealisation, it has been suggested that motherhood is a defining identity par excellence, and that the conflation of motherhood and womanhood means that mothers are constructed unitarily, and cease to be anything else (Richardson, 1993). Constructions of motherhood therefore involve both an exercise of power and a process of exclusion of identity. The experience of motherhood is characterised by 'relegation to silence, erasure, loss of subjectivity' (O'Barr, Pope & Wyer, 1990: 4). Constructions of motherhood as a labour of love render the workings of power invisible (Glenn, 1994). Oakley (1980; 1993) has argued that the primary loss involved in experiences of motherhood is a loss of identity and that dominant and individualised constructions isolate women, limiting their ability to seek alternatives or to resist dominant constructions of maternal 'normality'.

The idealisation and denigration of motherhood

If motherhood were characterised by happiness and fulfilment in actuality, and all mothers simply became the ideal, perhaps it would be unfair to critique idealisations of motherhood, since all social identities are likely to be predicated upon loss. Ideals of motherhood, however, are not 'real' and, like all idealisations, they only work if there is a corresponding denigration. Warner (1976) demonstrates this powerfully through an analysis of cultural representations of motherhood. The Virgin Mary represents the impossible ideal: serene, selfless and virgin pure. No other woman can be as good a mother as she. A more contemporary example, the Statue of Liberty, larger than life and giving birth to an entire nation, is a 'mother of mercy' and freedom, representing all that is good (Warner, 1985: 11). Offsetting the idealisation, however, is a stream of representations of mothers as monsters (Warner, 1994), beginning perhaps with the progenitor of motherhood, the evil Eve, who was punished for her sins with reproductive pain (Warner, 1985). Such figures provide fantasies of motherhood, as well as enjoinments and warnings. The fantasy of Mother Theresa, altruistically mothering the world's children while never procreating herself, enjoins selfless motherhood. The fantasy of the hideous mother in the *Alien* films, whose rampant maternal instinct devours and destroys, placing the core of society at threat, reminds us just how dangerous mothers can be. The idealised and denigrated mothers may be separate in fantasy, but their existence implies an ambivalence towards motherhood as potentially both creative and destructive (Coward, 1997). Since no actual mother exists at either extreme, the individual mother always fails to live up to the ideal and is always in danger of becoming a monster.

Constructions of motherhood therefore set up binary oppositions. It could be suggested that motherhood is idealised, while mothers themselves are often denigrated. The state of motherhood is promoted to that of a holy institution, while mothers are often constructed as not living up to this ideal. Binary oppositions regarding motherhood seem to work in two ways: by constructing categories of 'normal' and 'deviant' motherhood and by the production of a set of technologies (e.g. childcare manuals, visits to doctors, psychological knowledge) that remind women of the ever-present threat that they will fail, and therefore become 'bad' mothers instead of 'normal' mothers.

'Normal' mothers

Binary constructions of motherhood construct different maternal figures with reference to moralising discourses that divide 'good' mothers from 'bad' mothers (Sandelowski, 1990). This reconstruction is supported by contradictory constructions of maternity. For example:

> [M]others are romanticized as life-giving, self-sacrificing, and forgiving, and demonised as smothering, overly involved, and destructive. They are seen as all-powerful – holding the fate of their children and ultimately the future of society in their hands – and as powerless – subordinated to the dictates of nature, instinct, and social forces beyond their ken (Glenn, 1994: 11).

Maternal success can thus turn at any point into maternal failure: the line between life-giving and smothering, self-sacrificing and overly involved is potentially invisible, and 'natural' motherhood (be it as a force of nature or subjected to natural forces) can easily metamorphose into unnatural, powerful into too powerful, instinctual into fickle. These broader constructions are linked to contradictions in social discourses 'between prescriptions about what mothers should do and assertions that there are no hard and fast rules about mothering and that childrearing should be an individual, private affair' (Phoenix & Woollett, 1991a: 7). Ussher (1989) argues that such contradictions, in conjunction with veneration of some responses to motherhood and censure of others, serve to marginalise identities and relationships not tied up with mother and family. Expectations that mothers should obey the prescriptions and that they should know how to mother are maintained and concretised through the circulation of particular kinds of knowledge, most notably through institutions of medicine and psychology.

Medical knowledge, institutions and practices have become increasingly influential in managing motherhood, most obviously in relation to pregnancy and childbirth. The medicalisation of childbearing constructs mothers as medical subjects divorced from their social context, in which pregnancy is the only relevant status and medical expertise ('doctor knows best') has become the only knowledge of value (Oakley, 1980). This prevails throughout motherhood. If one's child is sick, for example, or is having difficulty with eating or potty training, medical expertise is constructed as the golden standard. In these cases, too, the mother is potentially a medical subject, although her child is the patient, for she may be causing maladies through bad mothering.

Foucaultian approaches trace the ways in which motherhood has increasingly been policed through the medical gaze (Rúdólfsdóttir, 2000). The trend towards medicalisation has sanitised the experience of motherhood, positioned expertise firmly within the realm of the medical establishment and spawned a number of regulatory practices that serve to place women under surveillance. Pregnancy has become a matter of medical surveillance and has been transformed into an objective observable process (Young, 1990). Foucaultian approaches stress that such processes cannot easily be understood through the concept of oppressive power, but rather that institutional surveillance filters into subjectivity such that the surveillance of the self (the question of whether one feels oneself to be a 'good' mother) implicates the subject within a web of discourse (Foucault, 1975). Motherhood has been professionalised through the filtering of medicalisation into the subjectivity of mothers and into the broader social sphere (Woollett & Phoenix, 1991). Medicalisation often supports broader discourses regarding the secondary nature of a mother's identity. For example, constructions of the foetus as sacred simultaneously displace the mother and her body to the status of object, reinforcing the child as the subject of motherhood (Kaplan, 1992; 1994), and medical expertise reinforces the notion that the mother's health is only of importance insofar as it supports the health of the baby. The maternal body is constructed as either nourishing or threatening. The mother's mind, for medicine, is a useful resource, given the right information, but is dangerously prone to emotional instability and irrationality (Rúdólfsdóttir, 2000). Both mind and body become subject to expertise, and psychology has been central in producing knowledge about motherhood.

There is a vast quantity of literature on motherhood, much of it from developmental psychology and childcare manuals (Phoenix & Woollett, 1991a; Marshall, 1991). Psychology has developed a complex set of theories about motherhood, although much of it is based on 'common sense' notions linked to dominant constructions of motherhood (Phoenix & Woollett, 1991b). Similar to the medicalisation of motherhood, psychology has produced a body of expertise and a plethora of normative statements that produce and monitor motherhood (Woollett & Phoenix, 1991). Along with this, a vocabulary has developed, designed to describe motherhood, but often blaming and judging mothers. Surrey (1990: 84) reflects on the language of psychological case reports and produces the following impressive list:

'engulfing,' 'controlling,' 'intrusive,' 'enmeshed,' 'seductive,' 'over-protective,' or, on the other hand, 'narcissistic,' 'critical,' 'cold,' 'unavailable,' 'unempathic,' 'distant,' 'depleted,' 'ineffective,' or 'depriving'.

Many of these words, such as 'symbiosis' or 'fusion', apply specifically to mothers and contribute to a pathologisation of motherhood as always potentially psychologically unhealthy (Caplan, 1990). The vocabulary exists together with guidelines about how to be a healthy mother producing psychologically healthy children, widely produced and consumed through childcare manuals, women's magazines and television programmes. Women have access to an enormous amount of psychological advice against which they can measure their adequacy as mothers.

Categories of deviance

Psychologised and medicalised constructions of motherhood are directed towards mothers (and potential mothers) everywhere. Phoenix and Woollett (1991a) suggest that motherhood is constructed as universally valued, but only as long as the mother fits normative stereotypes. Mothers classified as 'deviant', however, are constructed specifically around the source of the deviance. If the mother is too young (Phoenix, 1991); too old (Berryman, 1991); or is not white, middle class and in a stable heterosexual relationship (Walkerdine, 1984), this value unravels. Mothers may be deemed deviant because they have chosen an 'inappropriate' partner, as in lesbian motherhood (Pollack, 1990), or are single and have failed to choose a partner at all (Woodward, 1997). Constructions of motherhood as instinctive and innate set up other kinds of binaries. Childless women may be constructed as bad mothers, whether their childlessness is voluntary (Landa, 1990) or due to infertility (Sandelowski, 1990), and the myth of the wicked stepmother continues to exclude stepmothers from 'real' motherhood (Salwen, 1990). Wegar (1997) demonstrates the inescapability of constructions of deviance, analysing how clinical adoption literature depicts both birth and adoptive mothers as potentially bad mothers. 'Deviant' motherhood is therefore constructed by exclusion, leaving the category endlessly flexible and able to incorporate new types of motherhood. These constructions are, of course, not static and have received considerable revision in response to social change. Woodward (1997) traces reconstructions from the norm of the caring, stay-at-home mother to the more contemporary 'independent mother' who, balancing home and career, becomes a role model for her children. She notes, however, that this mother is also a fantasy figure, resisting previous constructions of deviancy, but consequently setting up a new ideal.

'Deviant' mothers are also potentially those who are demographically different to the Western (or Northern) norm. African-American mothers, for example, have been constructed either as custodians of a 'special bond' with their babies (Greene, 1990) or as reproductively uncontrollable due to their unrestrained sexuality (Solinger, 1994). The majority of critical theorising, however, has been conducted with a white and Western mother in mind (Phoenix & Woollett, 1991a). Featherstone (1997) notes that feminist interest in motherhood has arisen at least partly because of the perceived crisis regarding the breakdown of the Western nuclear family. This implies that the motivation for politicising motherhood, and not only the object of study, is assumed to be located in the Western world. Theorists have stressed that motherhood is culturally and historically constituted (Glenn, 1994), and some work has been done in this regard. Badinter (1981), for example, provides an historical analysis of French motherhood in order to argue that the 'maternal instinct' is mystical and mythical. Scheper-Hughes (1992) similarly argues that aspects of maternal indifference among Brazilian women, as well as changes in the value of motherhood and children, are linked to cultural, political and economic factors very different to those found in the West. Mothers in the developing world, however, remain under-researched and are presumed to be exotic.

Deconstructing motherhood

It is clear that the category of motherhood is culturally and historically constructed, is political and supports gendered power relations. It has been suggested that idealisations of motherhood both define and deny, and are accompanied by corresponding denigrations that create binary categories and contradictions. These feed into particular institutions, including medicine, psychology and political institutions. It should perhaps be added that feminism represents another institution that has constructed motherhood and has drawn upon ideals of motherhood as a key site of debate. The 'difference–equality knot' (Glenn, 1994: 22) – the debate concerning whether women are different from or equal to men – has been most vividly played out around the maternal body, and motherhood has become a major site of contestation in feminist theory. Chesler (1990) cites the inhumanity of feminists to one another as an example of the broader inhumanity of women towards women. In this way, maternity continues to be constructed within power relations.

Broader constructions hold implications for experiences of motherhood, but the task of deconstruction cannot necessarily account for the profound importance of motherhood to women. Motherhood may be idealised, denigrated and linked to institutions, but in the realm of experience, it 'is both a very ordinary thing to do and utterly extraordinary ... it brings emotional intensity and banality in equal measure' (Innes, 1995 in Woodward, 1997: 242). If motherhood is constructed within power relations, why do women feel such profound emotion about motherhood? Are constructions of idealisation and denigration converted into experience? These questions offer an opening for consideration of motherhood from a psychoanalytic perspective.

JOCASTA'S TALE

Of all the fantasies explored by psychoanalytic theory, the girl's fantasy of becoming a mother is the one wish that can actually come true. Miraculously and mysteriously, the wish to have a baby is turned into a reality. There is, of course, a difference between the original fantasy and the actual experience, partly because the woman is no longer a girl and partly because the experience of motherhood, mediated by so many unexpected factors and feelings, does not give the simple satisfaction of desire imagined during girlhood. Nonetheless, this is a rare instance where the miracle actually materialises.

Motherhood is given a special status in mainstream psychoanalysis, but not for this reason. The mother is seen as a primary and primal figure, but often a figure of danger and blame. Psychoanalysis routinely constructs the mother as secondary to the child and overlays her with fantasies similar to those it attributes to the infant. Psychoanalysis is commonly critiqued as mother-blaming, to the extent that both professionals and mothers themselves have internalised a pervasive tendency to seek blame first within the mother (Parker, 1995). The theory has had a profound influence on constructions of motherhood, but, it is fair to say, has also recognised motherhood as powerful and has offered a sustained account of the complexity of human experience. Psychoanalytic theory is potentially useful in understanding the mother's experience of motherhood (rather than the child's experience of motherhood) when psychoanalysis takes maternal subjectivity as its focus.

In mainstream psychoanalytic readings of the Oedipal drama, Oedipus is the subject to be analysed and understood. Stimmel (2004) refocuses attention on the tale, offering a psychoanalytic understanding of Jocasta as a mother longing for her son. She argues that Jocasta represents the hyperbole of normal maternal development and subjectivity, the 'pathological caricature of everywoman' (Stimmel, 2004: 1177). Attempting to understand Jocasta's subjectivity invokes taboos of incest and infanticide and situates these within maternal love and grief:

It is easy to forget that Jocasta did not just bed Oedipus; earlier, she tried to kill him in infancy. The stage is set for Jocasta remeeting her son at the intersection of her infantile desires and her maternal longings; a guilty, heartbroken mother longing for her lost child (Stimmel, 2004: 1182).

The child's wish for a baby is different from, although interlaced with, the mother's desires, because the subject has changed from child to mother. What is Jocasta's tale? What are her hopes and fears, conflicts and fantasies?

Recently, some psychoanalysts have turned their attention to the mother as subject, understanding motherhood itself as a psychodynamic event. This has been influenced by early psychoanalytic writers aiming specifically at understanding the transition to motherhood[1] and by psychoanalytic feminism, which uses psychoanalytic concepts to understand the relations and divisions between masculinity and femininity, and 'the making of a lady' (Mitchell, 1974), as well as interest in the role of motherhood in the social reproduction of gender (e.g. Chodorow, 1978; Dinnerstein, 1977).

Psychoanalytic work on motherhood is based on case studies and extensive interviews with mothers, in an attempt to explore psychodynamic aspects of subjectivity. In particular, there is agreement among recent writers that the period from pregnancy until shortly after birth marks a dramatic increase in psychodynamic activity, fantasy and conflicts (e.g. Parker, 1995; Raphael-Leff, 1993), particularly around the birth of the first child (Breen, 1975). The majority of this work (with the notable exception of Parker [1995]) focuses on pregnancy and motherhood during infancy, although these experiences are not necessarily confined to early motherhood.

These psychoanalytic writers tend to construct motherhood in terms of opportunity for the woman rather than damage to the child. For example:

The birth of a baby ... offers an opportunity for a woman to work through internal conflicts and relationships, to modify her perception of herself and others, and integrate this new experience so that she will not be the same after birth as she was before (Birksted-Breen, 2000: 17).

Birksted-Breen contrasts this developmental approach, which outlines normal, expected psychodynamic developmental processes of pregnancy,

1   For example, Deutsch (1945); Benedek (1959); Bibring et al. (1961a; 1961b); and Horney (1967).

to what she calls the hurdle approach (Breen, 1975), in which pregnancy is understood as a temporary state of abnormality to be overcome.

Developmental theories generally suggest that the psychodynamic experience of pregnancy is divided into three phases in line with the three trimesters, although there is some disagreement as to whether the birth of a child marks entry into a separate psychological state or whether it is continuous and part of the same developmental phase. Birksted-Breen (2000), for example, argues that the first phase of pregnancy is characterised by excitement and pride, but also by misgiving, conflict and withdrawal into the self, and by particular preoccupation with the symbolic division between inside and outside. In the second phase, fantasies and conflicts become more specifically related to the baby, and often evoke issues in relation to the woman's own mother. The task of this phase, then, is to negotiate relationships between self and other. The last phase of pregnancy is characterised by issues of separation and loss, retention and expulsion, and increased fear of the links between birth and death. The phase after birth sees the return of issues of life and death, but in a different form. In this phase, loss is connected to loss of pregnancy, loss of the fantasy baby and loss of identity. The usefulness of this and other models is that they provide a normative understanding of the conflicts of motherhood, which are able to formulate powerful feelings, defences and fantasies, as productive and not necessarily pathological. The woman's ability to mother, then, depends on the ways in which such conflicts are negotiated, rather than on the turgid nature of the conflicts per se (Parker, 1995).

Developmental views of motherhood shift focus from the baby to the mother, suggesting that becoming a mother prompts a number of conflicts and challenges through which the mother's identity is reworked (Breen, 1975; Raphael-Leff, 1993). Similarly, psychodynamic focus on understanding the conflicts, desires, fears and fantasies of mothers – the experience of motherhood – takes the mother and her subjectivity as the primary subject, thereby subverting the typical psychodynamic focus on the baby. Quite contrary to constructions of maternal bliss and selflessness, the mother's subjectivity is understood as complex and conflictual. When asked what struck them most about the experience of becoming a mother, Breen's (1975) respondents most often mentioned the miraculous nature of creating a new baby. The second common response cited the terror of childbirth. From the beginning of motherhood, then, there is a collision of unbelievable creativity and terrifying danger. Raphael-Leff (2000a) suggests that the experience of pregnancy, with two bodies in one, is frankly bizarre, and that a new baby is both compelling and disturbing:

> [E]xposure to the naked emotions, smell, feel, sound and suck of a tiny infant leaking primal matter from every orifice can be intensely arousing, particularly at a time when the caregiver feels hypersensitive and vulnerable. The compelling nature of close contact with a newborn is both insidious and most immediate ... its unmediated impact [may burst] an internal dam, with eruption of inexplicable feelings – of wild passions, poignant yearning, inarticulate dread, rage or despair – and in an attempt to cope with the threat of breakthrough anxieties, correspondingly primitive defences are mobilised to shore up internal barriers (Raphael-Leff, 2000b: 60).

Here Raphael-Leff describes the possibility of being overwhelmed by the immediacy of motherhood. It has been suggested that powerful fantasies, feelings and defences are, at least to some extent, endemic to experiences of early and later motherhood (Bradley, 2000; Parker, 1995). This is partly connected to idealised expectations of the joys of motherhood, which inevitably turn to disillusionment (Mills, 1997) and disappointment (Steiner, 1997). Motherhood offers opportunities for reparation and new beginnings (Bradley, 2000), but also involves multiple losses (Parker, 1995), including the loss of pregnancy and the loss of the fantasy baby (Mintzer et al., 2001). Early motherhood, in particular, is characterised by powerful fantasies and dreams (Stern, 1995; Raphael-Leff, 1993; Birksted-Breen, 2000), linked to fantasies about whether one's body has produced something good or bad (Breen, 1989).

From birth, motherhood also involves an ongoing process of separation and differentiation that is crucial in order to break the projections of maternal idealisation, but is nonetheless painful and involves a process of mourning (Pines, 1997; Steiner, 1997). The mother has to move from infantile fantasies of magical procreation in order to undo fusion and thereby allow the creativity of difference (Mariotti, 1997). This creative process is simultaneously one of loss and release, continually transforming identities of motherhood (Parker, 1995).

Kleinian concepts of splitting and projection have been usefully extended to provide an understanding of the mother's internal world. It has been suggested that objects, including her own mother and her baby, are incorporated into the mother's internal world and represent parts of herself. This has led Raphael-Leff (1989; 1993) to develop the 'Placental Paradigm', in which mother and baby are in dynamic relation to one another within the mother's mind, each potentially constructed as good or bad and evoking corresponding emotions and defences. Raphael-Leff (1989; 1993) explores various configurations of good/bad mother and baby, usefully foregrounding that the mother can feel her baby and/or herself as either good or bad – that this is an expected psychodynamic process in which badness and goodness reside. This presents a potential challenge to social idealisations of motherhood in which everything is always good unless there is something actually wrong with the mother.

It is also useful to consider the Placental Paradigm, because changes in its formulation may suggest some difficulties with comprehending the subjectivity of the mother herself. In an earlier formulation, Raphael-Leff (1989) describes four possible configurations:

1. Safe/good (nourishing) mother and safe/good (sustaining) baby;
2. Safe/good (bountiful) mother and dangerous/bad (parasitic) baby;
3. Dangerous/bad (polluting) mother and safe/good (innocent) baby;
4. Dangerous/bad (harmful) mother and dangerous/bad (harmful) baby.

This formulation suggests that the fantasised mother and baby represented in the mother's internal world are conceptualised in different forms and either prompt a consolidation (2 & 3) or a dismantling (1 & 4) of defensive barriers between mother and baby. It also suggests a framework for understanding the interaction between mother and baby within the mother's subjectivity. What this model does not include is an integrated, non-split position in which mother and baby are both good and bad. This emphasis on disintegration is echoed in Raphael-Leff's (1989: 28) definition that 'having a baby means contagious exposure to primitive experiences'. The emphasis is on contagion rather than on the coexistence of both good and bad.

This overemphasis on split aspects of motherhood seems to be addressed in a later reformulation of the Placental Paradigm (Raphael-Leff, 1993: 53):

Mother	Baby	Psychic interchange
±	±	Ambivalent coexistence
+	+	Idealised exchange
+	–	Mother's barrier against 'parasitic' baby
–	+	Mother feels dangerous to vulnerable baby
+/–	0	Bipolar conflict; good/bad splitting; baby = non-entity

This reformulation starts with the possibility of 'ambivalent coexistence', in which mother and baby are both good and bad. Interestingly, however, something else drops off the model: there is no longer the possibility that both mother and baby are experienced as bad (i.e. no –/–: no dangerous/ bad mother and dangerous/bad baby). If the mother experiences herself as bad (indicated by the minus sign), the baby is either seen to be experienced as good (+) or as non-existent (0). Put differently, a bad baby can only have a good mother. In the first model, babies and mothers have to be either good or bad; when ambivalence is allowed in, bad baby and bad mother are limited and kept separate.

There may have been many reasons for the shift in this model. Here, I would like to suggest that the shift tells us something about the discomfort evoked when comprehending maternal fantasies and subjectivity. In the first formulation, maternal subjectivity is understood as either good or bad. When ambivalence enters, too much badness becomes incomprehensible. This is usefully considered in light of Parker's (1995: 94) argument that:

> Mothers respond to the element of hatred in their maternal ambivalence with a similar sense of loss of an internal good object. This may provoke either persecutory guilt (the problem is he's a bad baby) or depressive guilt (the problem is I'm a bad mother).

Parker argues that maternal ambivalence is unavoidable and expected, and is also highly creative and useful. Part of the difficulty, however, is that mothers do not expect to feel ambivalent. Parker suggests that the bad baby and the bad mother are imagined as a result of different kinds of guilt, but in both cases in response to maternal hatred. It is possible to build from this a somewhat more fluid understanding of bad and good babies and mothers within maternal subjectivity. Persecutory guilt, for Klein, resides in the paranoid schizoid position, and depressive guilt in the depressive position. The two are in relation to one another: depressive guilt is linked to the desire for reparation after a persecutory projection. In this sense, it may be that the mother experiences the baby and herself as bad, but, given social idealisations of motherhood, she is likely to experience herself as bad *because* she has experienced the baby as bad. She is a bad mother for daring to think that her baby is anything but good. Reconceptualised in this way, the bad baby is the result of an emotion or projection, whereas the feeling of being a bad mother is a punishment for that emotion or projection. If the baby is fantasised as bad, it is felt to be so because of the mother.

Thinking about the baby and the mother as internal objects within the mother's mind is useful when something actually does go wrong, e.g. when the baby dies (Etchegoyen, 1997; Piontelli, 2000), is handicapped (Sinason, 1992; Birksted-Breen, 2000) or is born with a birth defect (Mintzer et al., 2001) – or is potentially HIV-positive. Psychoanalytic consideration of these circumstances suggests that if something is actually wrong with the baby, the mother is likely to feel responsible, as if she has given the bad parts of herself to her baby. Related guilt about what she has done and, if a baby dies, survivor guilt that she has survived, are common, while something 'wrong' with the baby is often seen as a narcissistic injury. If the baby really is bad in some way, it is because of the mother.

These different formulations suggest the threats involved in feeling like a bad mother and also suggest the complexity of maternal subjectivity from a psychodynamic perspective. The smoothed versions of motherhood, so hoped for in the social imagination, are illustrated instead through psychodynamic conflict and creativity. Placing Jocasta at centre stage shifts understandings of relationships by employing similar psychodynamic concepts to those applied to the baby.

The spectral mother

Both the social constructions and psychodynamic experiences of motherhood evoke opposites: of power and powerlessness, idealisation and denigration, birth and death, good and bad. Social constructions tend to construct motherhood as either/or, in contrast to experiences of motherhood, which are both/and. Parker (1995: x) emphasises that social representations of motherhood also inform experiences of motherhood in ways that reinforce the split between good and bad:

> Cultural and public representations of good and bad mothering interact with the unique, personal, private, emotional meanings mothering has for a woman. Mothers both reproduce and resist assumptions of what it means to mother – but those assumptions cannot be escaped ... A deeper understanding of the production, purpose and prohibition of maternal ambivalence can enable mothers

(and others) to see that most mothers are neither as 'bad' as we fear, nor as 'good' as we desire.

Perhaps, then, understanding the 'joys of motherhood', with all their connotations of social expectation and personal ambivalence, involves undoing the split between good and bad. In order to do this, motherhood must be understood from the perspective of both the mother and the baby. The invisibility of motherhood needs to be undone.

Part of the difficulty of this task is that everybody has experienced a mother, but only mothers have experienced motherhood. Motherhood is partly elusive because it is a dual position, of being a mother as well as of having been mothered, and empathy is strongest for the child's experience of the mother. Entangled in experience is the dominance of patriarchal culture in defining motherhood, which, in Kaplan's (1992: 40) words, presents a challenge to 'honouring the mother's subjectivity, the mother's voice'.

Kaplan, along with Kristeva and Sprengnether, represent three examples of feminist theorist who have explicitly argued for the importance of acknowledging the mother's subjectivity and voice. Although others have written about the maternal position, these three theorists have been chosen as illustrative, because, in each case, there are points where the focus on the mother fails or slips in the face of the needs of the child. Through examining these moments, their work can be used to illustrate the elusiveness of the maternal position, suggesting, perhaps, that focus on motherhood from the mother's perspective is slippery, because the figure of the mother evokes powerful fantasies and anxieties.

Kaplan (1992: 40) argues as follows:

Many theorists of motherhood ... end up looking from the child position. That slippage from talking about the mother to talking from the child's perspective seems endemic to research in this area, and is itself revealing of the instability of the mother construct.

Kristeva is one of the theorists that Kaplan explores to demonstrate this slippage. In Kristeva's early work, the maternal perspective is celebrated as subversive, because it holds a unique meaning. Her concept of the semiotic attempts to remove maternal (and infantile) experience from patriarchy and to imply a uniqueness to the maternal body. In her essay 'Stabat mater' (Kristeva, 1986), she explicitly includes her own maternal voice in the text. In one column talking academically about motherhood, in another talking poetically about her own maternal experience, she insists on the inclusion of maternal subjectivity in the exploration of maternal representations.

In contrast, Kristeva's (1982) theory of abjection positions the mother very differently. According to Kristeva, the abject turns the stomach – it prompts gagging and retching. She includes examples such as the skin on the surface of milk, bodily waste or muck, or a corpse. The abject is frightening because it is neither fully inside nor fully outside the self, and therefore threatens the boundaries of 'me'. The abject does not signify death only because it is outside of signification: it '*show[s] me* what I permanently thrust aside in order to live' (Kristeva, 1982: 3) and therefore threatens to take 'me' with it.

At first glance, it seems that HIV-positive motherhood represents a contradiction, because HIV fits frighteningly into the category of the abject, but is actually inside the idealised maternal body. For Kristeva, however, there would be no contradiction: the maternal body is the original abject – the most frightening place where boundaries between self and (m)other cannot be maintained, and therefore threaten to annihilate. It is this shift that Kaplan comments upon: in her earlier theories, maternal subjectivity is primary. In her later theories, the focus is on the child's subjectivity. Through abjection, the mother's perspective is lost.

Ironically, Kaplan then seems to make a similar slip away from maternal subjectivity. She comments: 'Kristeva seems to be talking about the mother from the child perspective, whereas in the earlier work she tried to speak from the (impossible) mother position' (Kaplan, 1992: 43). Kaplan's argument is based on the importance of 'honour[ing] the mother's subjectivity' (Kaplan, 1992: 40). In her critique of Kristeva for failing to maintain this approach, she introduces one word, in brackets – 'impossible' – that invalidates the possibility of honouring the mother's subjectivity. She slips away from the mother's perspective, because in this moment it seems 'impossible'.

A third theorist to argue that the mother should be understood as subject rather than object is Sprengnether (1990). She argues that psychoanalytic theory has failed to comprehend the originary nature of maternity, focusing on her re-reading of Freud and other psychoanalytic theorists in search of the spectral mother.

Towards the end of her book, she notes the importance of understanding 'birth from the mother's point of view' (Sprengnether, 1990: 238). Immediately after this, her finale ends with analysis of a novel called *Housekeeping*. It is about two sisters, Ruth and Lucille, who have been orphaned by their mother's suicide and then looked after by their grandmother. When she too dies, they are cared for by eccentric Aunt Sylvie. Sprengnether is particularly interested in Ruth's internal voyage in search of her own conception. For example, she quotes and discusses Ruth's striking formulation that '[b]y some bleak alchemy what had been mere unbeing becomes death when life is mingled with it' (Sprengnether, 1990: 242).

Sprengnether analyses the story to stress her argument that the mother's body is originary. She does not comment, however, on the fact that she is no longer understanding 'birth from the mother's point of view'. The story can say nothing about the mother's point of view, because the mother is dead. Having committed suicide – perhaps the ultimate act of maternal selfishness – she can only be understood from the child's point of view, and only in relation to her evocation of both life and death.

These three shifts away from the mother towards the perspective of the child do not only reveal 'the instability of the mother construct' (Kaplan, 1992: 40). Maternal subjectivity is undone because of the mother's associations with abjection (Kristeva), impossibility (Kaplan) and death (Sprengnether). In addition to the idealisations and denigrations that have recurred throughout this chapter, it is suggested that the mother's position is elusive because of these associations. If this is the 'ordinary' mother, what does it mean to be an HIV-positive mother, in which the impossibility, abjection and death associated with motherhood are compounded by HIV, with its own abjection, impossibility and death?

MOTHERHOOD IN SOUTH AFRICA

Contemporary South Africa is a mélange of different cultures and images. With 11 official languages and an array of foreign influence, both historically and currently, diversity is probably the most defining characteristic of South African society. It is informed by past and present, and is both urban and rural, developed and developing, rich and poor. South African mothers draw upon a range of cultural practices, although many of the ideals and deprecations discussed above apply to them across cultural locations. Discussion here will focus largely on black women, because they represent the majority and because the stories of black women form the focus of this book.[2] Constructions of African motherhood will be explored in relation to history and culture, although it would be misleading to suggest that such influences have determined experiences of motherhood or that 'African culture' is a static phenomenon.

Scholarship on African motherhood also produces a far from static picture, echoing the contestations regarding the nature of motherhood found in international literature. As Kruger (2006) points out, very little research has been conducted on South African motherhood, particularly in relation to maternal experience. The perspectives of contemporary South African mothers themselves are not well documented, apart from a few studies, most of which examine the experiences of white middle-class South African mothers. Examples include Daniels (2004); Frizelle & Hayes (1999); Jeannes & Shefer (2004); Kruger (2003); and Lesch & Kruger (2005).

These studies suggest the centrality of notions of motherhood as selfless, natural and ideal, although this construction is also resisted and overturned by actual mothers.

2   For a definition of how this book uses the term 'black women', see chapter 1, note 1.

Daniels (2004: 1) argues that the general trend in South African research has been to portray black mothers, particularly poor mothers, as helpless victims, 'with little or no control over their lives; as objects to be bartered for by men; to be invested similar to property'. Even this view, however, is contested, particularly through historical studies tracing the centrality of motherhood in the political development of South Africa (Walker, 1990; 1995). The resourcefulness of mothers in the face of poverty and absent men has also received attention (Daniels, 2004). In relation to black mothers, two very different images are persuasively offered: the image of the strong mother and that of the mother oppressed in terms of both gender and race.

Historical studies of motherhood have focused largely on the period from colonialism onwards, although it has been noted that prior constructions of motherhood remain important for black women, particularly regarding the value placed on fertility and the relative power motherhood offers to women (Walker, 1995). It has been suggested that cultural practices and beliefs in relation to motherhood have been transformed by colonialism, where Christian and traditional belief systems began to interact (Guy, 1990). Traditional beliefs and practices remain important, but to different degrees for different people. The content of traditional beliefs and practices has also shifted in relation to competing belief systems and historical change. Colonialism and, later, urbanisation and Westernisation have strongly influenced African conceptions of motherhood, and historical analyses have suggested that Christian notions of motherhood were dominant from the mid-twentieth century (Walker, 1991), although these have merged with African formulations rather than subsuming them completely (Walker, 1990).

Constructions of motherhood during apartheid have also merged with both Western and traditional formulations. Motherhood was idealised on both sides of the apartheid struggle. Afrikaner nationalism included the revered concept of the *volksmoeder* ('mother of the nation'), who was dependent on, but supportive of her men (Brink, 1990), and responsible for producing and maintaining Afrikaner culture (Du Toit, 2003).

The *volksmoeder* was a key figure in the moral justification of Afrikaner nationalism. Interestingly, political rhetoric today also refers to the 'mother of the nation', although this mother is constructed as African and not Afrikaans. This suggests the centrality of the concept – and the centrality of motherhood – to both nationalist projects.

On the other side of the struggle, African women often organised politically around their identities as mothers (Walker, 1991). Mothers, as custodians of culture and of future leaders, were understood as central to the fight against apartheid. Indeed, it has been suggested that while motherhood was central to the political project for both black and white women, white women tended to be portrayed as more passive and home-centred, while black women had a more active and stronger voice (Walker, 1995).

Women activists, however, were not constructed unproblematically. Primarily intervening against apartheid as mothers, since this was their most legitimate access to politics (Walker, 1990), women were often curtailed in their activities *because* they were mothers. Apartheid police and prison guards taunted female activists for failing to be proper women: 'you are an unnatural woman, an unnatural mother' (Ross, 2003: 65). Similarly, fellow male activists accused women involved in the struggle of 'being inadequate mothers and betraying cultural ideals of motherhood' (Ross, 2003: 146). As one of Ross's (2003: 147) respondents says, 'they said we were acting against our culture in teaching those children politics. They said we were wrong. They told me I was betraying my culture. They used culture against us.'

Attempts by women to fight for political freedom were thus limited on both sides and were connected to both racial prejudice and patriarchal discourse. Indeed, many women were fighting for both gender and racial equality (Ross, 2003). Motherhood gave them the legitimacy to fight and was the basis upon which political involvement was rejected. Walker has moderated her initial historical analysis that female activism was essentially conservative because of its reliance on maternalist discourse (Walker, 1982), moving towards a recognition that women were constrained by, but also found political agency through maternity (Walker, 1990).

Motherhood was a key site of identity struggle during apartheid; it was also profoundly affected by apartheid. The movement of black people was tightly monitored through complex systems of pass laws, delineated 'homelands' and the migrant labour system. The migrant labour system encouraged young men to seek work in urban settings, leaving families in designated rural 'homelands'. These systems undermined traditional family structures (Duncan & Rock, 1997); resulted in men having families in both urban and rural areas; and, as the gender divide lessened and more women sought work in urban areas, hastened urbanisation (Guy, 1990). While traditional values continue to be placed on motherhood, female-headed households have increased in both urban and rural settings (Pick & Obermeyer, 1996), placing added responsibility on mothers. This move has been variously interpreted as constraining mothers even further and also as a situation in which mothers accessed more autonomy, control over labour and freedom from men (Daniels, 2004).

Perhaps based upon earlier colonial notions of African women as hyperfertile and sexually dangerous (Upton, 2001) and white fears about black population growth (Kaufman, 2000), apartheid family planning programmes specifically directed at the black population were designed to limit fertility. These programmes were legitimately perceived as racist, but did not go as far as to involve involuntary sterilisation (Potts & Marks, 2001). Apartheid policies therefore directly intervened in reproductive decisions and raised suspicion. This suspicion remains today, at least to some extent, and has posed a challenge in the fight against HIV (with condoms perceived to be 'white' and 'dangerous'), as well as continuing to limit the reproductive freedom of black women. South Africa's history has therefore changed and modified constructions of motherhood between and within groups.

Despite historical shifts and increasing diversity, African motherhood remains a central, even defining, identity. 'Mother' and 'woman', for example, are frequently considered to be interchangeable terms (Walker, 1982), and the word 'mother' is a compliment as well as a descriptor. Mothers are seen as custodians of culture, responsible for keeping it alive, and motherhood is respected and honoured (James & Busia, 1994; Nhlapo, 1991). To reject one's mother, potentially, is to reject the 'African way of thinking' (Long & Zietkiewicz, 2006). African motherhood is idealised, and also holds consequences for the deviant. Schlyter (in Potts & Marks, 2001: 204) describes Southern African respondents' fears of not being able to claim identities of motherhood:

> The nightmare of the girls was to be barren .... Barren women were not only pitied, but also seen as lacking some of the qualities of real women ... a boy told me that his stepmother was barren; he expected me to assume that she was wicked.

The dominant cultural construction is that mothers are 'real' women, and that mothers themselves are secondary to their children.

Although motherhood is highly valued, traditional beliefs are patriarchal and not matriarchal, and men have traditionally been understood as responsible for reproductive decisions (Potts & Marks, 2001). A paradox of motherhood in African society is that black women are revered for their fertility and restricted because of it (Nhlapo, 1991). This is evident in traditional practices, which are still observed, although to varying degrees. The ability to produce a child is highly esteemed, to the extent that it may be necessary for a woman to produce a child in order to get married (Walker, Reid & Cornell, 2004). When a couple decide to marry, the man's family pays *lobola* (bridewealth) to the family of his bride-to-be. Through this transaction, the woman is expected to move families, and any children will belong to her husband's family as well as to herself (Guy, 1990). A woman who does not produce children as expected may face 'grave hardship for breaking the unwritten stipulations of the marital contract and may consequently be abandoned emotionally, socially and financially' (Harrison & Montgomery, 2001: 312). Infertility is on the rise (Potts & Marks, 2001), partly because of HIV, although the trend predates the rise of the epidemic (Harrison & Montgomery, 2001), and cultural issues connected to reproduction are consequently gaining importance. A number of reasons have been suggested for the rise of infertility, including that it is one way for women to maintain control in a society where violence against women is extremely high (Naidoo, 2002).

As yet, research has focused predominantly on involuntary infertility; the women interviewed for this book often did not want to bear more children for fear of transmitting HIV to their children, but, in the absence of disclosure of their HIV status, found this position difficult to support, given cultural idealisations of motherhood. Cultural and historical constructions of motherhood have a bearing on these and other decisions mothers are faced with on a daily basis.

Characterising South African motherhood, then, is a task that necessarily emphasises the impact of mothering ideologies, originating in both Western and African contexts and developing in relation to both, but maintaining very particular constructions of mothers as somehow different from others. The values placed on motherhood, contested though these may be, return 'motherhood' to a reified concept that is portrayed much more clearly than it is lived.

CONCLUSION

This chapter has explored the ways in which motherhood is constructed in theory and in the South African context. Feminist work has attempted to reposition motherhood at centre stage in order to suggest the extent to which one's perspective needs to (and often fails to) change in order to see maternity through the mother's eyes. Mainstream psychoanalysis has often failed to take this perspective, instead portraying maternity as problematic and originary of later conflicts. The psychoanalytic writers explored above, who have moved the mother from the periphery to centre stage, offer a very different understanding of maternity as developmental, complex and far from passive. Constructions of South African motherhood have shifted historically and culturally, but continue to be idealised in ways that limit, but also fail to encapsulate, experiences of motherhood.

4. Finding the HIV-positive Mother

Finding the HIV-positive mother between constructions of motherhood and of HIV and between the social and psychodynamic resonances of the two identities involves finding a multitude of positions, identities, meanings and emotions rather than finding a fixed and definable entity. This chapter explores possible processes of finding HIV-positive motherhood, taking two very different approaches. Firstly, the chapter explores the kind of HIV-positive mother who has been 'found' in the scientific literature and critically examines the ways in which this figure has been constructed, socially and perhaps also unconsciously. Secondly, the chapter suggests a possible framework for understanding HIV-positive motherhood as lying *between* inner and outer reality. This section draws on the psychodynamic and the discursive as a prelude to the chapters that follow, in which interview data is directly explored.

FINDING THE HIV-POSITIVE MOTHER IN THE SCIENTIFIC IMAGINATION

Reading photographs of HIV-positive mothers involves looking for social discourses and psychodynamic meanings regarding the fantasies hidden in the representations. Studies on HIV-positive motherhood can be similarly read. If women are invisible in the AIDS epidemic, mothers – ironically constructed as a separate category to women – are considerably more so. This is despite the common practice of countries estimating prevalence rates from statistics gathered at antenatal clinics. There is remarkably little research or social commentary on HIV-positive motherhood, and the research that does exist constructs mothers only in relation to the harm HIV-positive mothers could potentially cause their babies. Zivi (1998: 49) notes that when mothers do become the object of focus, this trend serves to 'demonize pregnant women, scapegoating them for perinatal transmission of HIV, and coding them as irresponsible, irrational, uncaring mothers'. Somewhat more colourfully, Patton (1993: 175) suggests that when HIV-positive women 'are not vaginas waiting to infect men, they are uteruses, waiting to infect fetuses'. Part-objects defined by reproductive organs, damage and infectiousness, mothers are constructed as an extremely problematic category.

It is striking that the ways in which HIV-positive mothers are spoken about, both in academic literature and in the public realm, are often characterised by either the idealisation of their status as mothers (and concomitant denial of the emotional pain involved in being HIV-positive) or by denigration through the identification of deficit. In attempting to establish whether HIV-positive mothers are either good or bad, it seems to be difficult to hold a more realistic position that they may be neither and both. It appears that, firstly, the actual experiences of mothers are not being given a voice, and secondly, the research conducted tends to be descriptive rather than theoretically rich.

While it would be unfair to minimise the importance of existing research on HIV-positive motherhood or to dismiss the quality of some of this work,

I will focus my critique on the claim that such research fails to take the HIV-positive mother as a subject in her own right. I will argue that obsessive measuring of the HIV-positive mother within this research indicates fears of the HIV-positive mother as destructive. While the research offers descriptors, it leaves us with little sense of what the experience of being an HIV-positive mother must be like. Some of the slips in the literature will be examined in order to prompt thoughts regarding the representation of HIV-positive mothers in the scientific imagination. If we examine some of these gaps and points of irrationality, we can see how the construction of motherhood either slips in contradictory or nonsensical ways or becomes general and vague. The themes of absence, death, guilt and abnormality subsequently emerge.

Research on HIV-positive motherhood is largely measurement based. Of the huge range of psychological variables available to researchers, very few find their way into research on HIV-positive mothers. Speculation of the reasons for this could be wide ranging, but the question of what HIV-positive mothers invoke in the popular imagination and the kind of panic they create in the scientific imagination (Squire, 1997) is a provocative one to pose. Existing research concerns itself with four focus areas: disclosure, incidence of psychiatric symptoms, coping and support, and parenting. Each will be discussed in relation to constructions of HIV-positive motherhood.

Perhaps it is impossible to answer the question of why research on HIV-positive mothers seems to slip away from the supposed object of study — the mothers themselves. One possible way of thinking about this is to use examples in the literature where the construction of motherhood seems to slip in contradictory and nonsensical ways, and then to ask how the 'HIV-positive mother' might be constructed within the scientific imagination. My method in doing this has been to read the literature with an eye open for places where the HIV-positive mother has seemed to break out of the objectivity and formality of scientific reporting and for places where irrational connections are made. Somewhat akin to Freud's ear for slips of the tongue, these examples have been read as containing possible hints towards understanding how the HIV-positive mother may be evocative. Four examples will be presented, in <u>this different font</u>, as a counterpoint to the 'rationality' of research on HIV-positive motherhood.

Disclosure

Studies of disclosure of HIV status are common in the broader HIV/AIDS literature, largely because disclosure is believed to limit the spread of the epidemic. The word 'disclosure' has become part of HIV discourse and is laden with associations of infection. Studies on motherhood have a somewhat different concern, focusing on disclosure between mother and child.

Studies have demonstrated that HIV-positive mothers seldom disclose their HIV status to their children (Salter Goldie, DeMatteo & King, 1997; Nöstlinger et al., 2004). Factors associated with non-disclosure include fear of losing social support, uncertainty regarding how to disclose, difficulties in planning for future care of their children (Murphy et al., 1999), fear that children would be unable to keep the information confidential or would be stigmatised themselves, and reluctance to contemplate their own deaths (Simoni et al., 2000).

When children themselves were HIV-positive, approximately 50 per cent of parents informed their children of their diagnosis (Lee & Johann-Liang, 1999; Murphy et al., 1999). This was in many cases prevented by similar factors to disclosure of maternal HIV status, but was also thought to be linked to cultural factors governing parenting practices and to maternal guilt (Lee & Johann-Liang, 1999). These findings suggest that children are frequently not told of their health status even after they become symptomatic.

HIV-positive mothers are the subjects of most disclosure studies, but it seems that it is often concern for children that motivates these studies. Siegel and Gorey (1994), for example, are concerned that *lack of disclosure* may lead to confusion, as well as feelings of responsibility and guilt in children, while Shaffer et al. (2001) are concerned that *disclosure* will lead to child behavioural problems and deterioration of the mother–child relationship.

Neither study is able to demonstrate that the authors' fears are well founded. Simoni et al. (2000) are similarly concerned with the impact of family secrets on children, while Armistead et al. (2001: 11) find that disclosure, 'contrary to expectation', is unrelated to the child's functioning.

This bind, reinforced by the research questions that are chosen, situates the HIV-positive mother as potentially bad if she does disclose, and bad if she doesn't. Further, disclosure seems to become a variable that is only measured for its presence or absence, rather than a conceptual tool for understanding the complexities involved in disclosing HIV status in the context of the mother–child relationship.

Lee and Johann-Liang (1999) study maternal disclosure. In their literature review, they acknowledge that maternal guilt may be a factor preventing disclosure. They then present the fairly low disclosure rates that they found in their study and, in their discussion section, list a number of reasons why disclosure may be difficult. 'For vertically transmitted HIV infection,' however, 'maternal guilt can be the only reason for withholding diagnosis from the child' (Lee & Johann-Liang, 1999: 43). This implies that if the child were infected by other means, mothers would have several reasons not to disclose, but if maternal guilt is present, it must clearly be the only reason. Indeed, this is a difficult reason to engage with, but the foregrounding of maternal guilt above and beyond everything else seems to be more an assumption of the authors than a demonstrated conclusion that they can justify through their findings. Maternal guilt eclipses the mother, leaving her with no thoughts other than of her own guilt. The thoughtful or worried mother is replaced by the guilty, withholding mother on the basis of no other criterion than her own HIV-positive status.

Incidence of psychiatric symptoms

Studies have found extraordinarily high levels of psychiatric diagnoses and psychological disturbance among HIV-positive mothers (e.g. Taylor, Amodei & Mangos, 1996). Diagnoses of depression and post-traumatic stress disorder are most common (Murphy et al., 1999), and the risk of depression seems to endure over time (Jones, Beach & Frehand, 2001). Lee and Rotheram-Borus (2001) demonstrate that parents who survived for a considerable length of time demonstrated higher levels of anxiety at the time of diagnosis, but a decrease in anxiety over time. Parents who died during their study, and were thus assumed to have progressed to AIDS-related illnesses, tended to have initially lower anxiety that increased over time. This indicates the link between psychiatric symptoms and mortality.

As with studies on disclosure, it seems that studies of psychiatric disturbance are at least partly interested in answering the question of whether HIV-positive mothers are potentially damaging to their children. Studies have compared mothers and children, finding that both HIV-positive mothers and their children are more likely to be depressed than HIV-negative mothers and their children (Biggar & Forehand, 1998; Forehand et al., 1998). Forsyth et al. (1996) found evidence of increased depression among children of HIV-positive mothers, but not increased anxiety. They did find, however, that anxiety increased when mothers were symptomatic. Murphy et al. (2002) note that depressed mothers were less able to perform daily tasks, resulting in children being more responsible for the household. Miles et al. (1997) are interested in maternal depression because of its potential implications that depressed mothers are less able to develop positive mother–infant relationships. All of these findings are important, but are specifically directed at identifying mothers who cause problems for their children.

The link between HIV status and psychiatric disturbance, however, is not always clear. It has been noted that depression is more likely if the father/partner is absent (Bennetts et al., 1999) and less likely if the woman discloses her status to her partner (Armistead et al., 1999). It has also been suggested that psychiatric disturbance is not necessarily HIV-related (Silver et al., 2003) and is most influenced by stress and social support (Mellins et al., 2000). Nonetheless, the titles of studies on psychiatric disturbance invariably foreground HIV-positive motherhood as the area of focus, implying a specific link between disturbance and this identity. Moreover, studies typically use samples of impoverished women, and often intravenous drug-using mothers, without always commenting on the implications of these factors for psychiatric disturbance. HIV becomes the overwhelming marker of identity, and the implication is that there is something about being an HIV-positive mother that is likely to drive one (and one's children) mad.

Miles et al. (1997) conduct a thorough study on 'personal, family and health-related correlates of depressive symptoms in mothers with HIV' (Miles et al., 1997: 23). In their literature review, they identify feelings of personal responsibility as a possible factor accounting for depression. Of their list of factors, this is the only one they do not include in their research design. While feelings of personal responsibility were not directly measured, two items on their stigma scale prompted this conclusion:

> It is interesting to note that the items with the highest mean scores on the scale were 'I feel ashamed' and 'I thought the illness was a punishment', supporting the view that mothers' perceptions of stigma may be related to lifestyle factors contributing to their illness (Miles et al., 1997: 30).

To attribute feelings of shame to lifestyle factors (i.e. real things that the woman has done to deserve shame) rather than to *feelings* of shame, a much more complex issue, seems again to indicate something about the way in which HIV-positive mothers are constructed, since this conclusion cannot be supported by the data. The assumption is that feelings of shame and retribution are causally linked to the woman's actions in reality, and that this is of importance to their status as mothers. Were the same expressions of shame and retribution to be made by mothers suffering from another terminal illness, they would be heard as expressions of emotion rather than admissions of responsibility.[1] Personal feelings of responsibility have been reinterpreted as

---

1   See Sontag's (1988) discussion of the ways in which AIDS is ascribed different meanings to other diseases such as cancer.

proof of personal responsibility. The HIV-positive mother, then, is constructed as a blameworthy object and thus as a legitimate carrier of guilt.

Coping and support

Studies focusing on coping and support tend to attempt a more fine-grained understanding of the experience of HIV-positive mothers, although these studies often tend to produce fairly obvious lists of conclusions. Prado et al. (2004) find that religion may have positive or negative consequences for coping. Heath and Rodway (1999) conclude that the psychosocial needs of HIV-positive women include help and support, financial help and recognition of the emotional impact of the diagnosis. Marcenko and Samost (1999) cite resources for coping as spirituality, the inner strength of the women, positive thinking and support from others. Rose and Clark-Alexander (1996) conclude, unsurprisingly, that HIV-positive mothers use all three of the coping mechanisms that they define, while Chalfin, Grus and Tomaszeski (2002) find that biological and foster mothers of HIV-positive children employ similar coping strategies. Van Loon (2000) believes that the only two issues troubling HIV-positive mothers are reunion with children removed from home and conflictual relationships with adult children. She adds that this is particularly the case among intravenous drug-using mothers. This rather narrow list illustrates the broader trend to portray mothers only in relation to their children. Similarly, Hough et al. (2003) are interested in the impact of maternal coping on the psychosocial adjustment of children, finding mixed results, despite their assertion that children of HIV-positive mothers are extremely vulnerable. It does appear, however, that worries about others may take precedence over worries about self (Rose & Clark-Alexander, 1996; DeMarco, Lynch & Board, 2002) and that HIV-positive mothers are primarily concerned with their children, through which they find meaning and hope (D'Auria, Christian & Shandor Miles, 2006; Shambley-Ebron & Boyle, 2006). HIV-positive women asked to identify their greatest worries identified concern regarding the health of their children and the future of their families (Manopaiboon et al., 1998). More textured and explanatory studies are clearly needed in this area.

Studies that propose to address the experiences of motherhood tend to be characterised by thin descriptions. Heath and Rodway (1999), for example, have a section entitled 'The experience of being HIV-positive'. This experience is summed up as a need to be listened to, a need for spirituality and a discussion of the experiences of older women mourning the deaths of their husbands. Surely there is more to the experience of being HIV-positive than this? Rose (1993, in Rose & Clark-Alexander, 1996: 44) describes the coping behaviours of HIV-positive women as 'prayer, cleaning house, sleeping, eating, and watching television'. These everyday activities do not capture the intricacy of the struggle to cope. In a similar vein, Van Loon (2000) states that HIV-positive mothers redefine motherhood in two (and by implication, only two) ways: by emphasising tasks that they are still able to perform when their health changes and by reframing motherhood as oversight of well-being when their children are in the care of others. There is undoubtedly more to motherhood than this.

A British study (Barrett & Victor, 1994), emotively entitled 'We just want to be a normal family', appraised HIV hospital services. The title, which is clearly a quotation from a research participant, implies that the participant is imploringly wishing to be normal, but, being HIV-positive, is not. The HIV-positive person is thus constructed as enduringly abnormal. Towards the end of the article, the authors place this quotation in context. The research participant is explaining that she does not want to utilise voluntary support groups, because HIV 'hasn't taken over our lives. We just want to be a normal family' (Barrett & Victor, 1994: 428). The context makes it clear that the participant is using this statement in an effort to resist constructions of abnormality, and not as an acceptance of abnormality, as the title of the article implies. Thus, where the participant proclaims normality, the title seems to imply its impossibility. The assignation of abnormality seems to reside in the challenge of HIV to the sanctity of the family. Within an empathically written article arises the rupture of defect and aberration.

Parenting

Studies aiming to measure the parenting efficacy of HIV-positive mothers appear to be somewhat more problematic than studies of other issues. The motivating factor of such studies is to establish whether HIV-positive mothers are bad parents. The findings of different studies tend to be contradictory. Studies also do not always control for maternal drug use. This may be a potential confounding variable in parenting efficacy, since it is unclear in many studies whether findings regarding parenting efficacy are related to HIV status or drug use. Studies on parenting also predominantly focus on child psychosocial adjustment (Family Health Project Research Group, 1998; Pilowsky, Wissow & Hutton, 2000), taking insufficient account of the effects of often multiple loss children experience and implying that lack of adjustment is a sole function of having an HIV-positive mother. The assumption that HIV-positive mothers must be bad mothers is demonstrated in Hale et al.'s (1999) attempt to test an assessment tool for maternal emotional involvement on HIV-positive mothers. Although they cite Black, Nair and Harrington's (1994) study that concludes that HIV-positive mothers are more emotionally involved, they attribute their mixed results to problems with the instrument rather than problems with their assumption that they have chosen a group of 'bad' mothers.

Some studies seem to demonstrate that parenting is adversely affected by maternal HIV-positive diagnosis. There is concern that children of HIV-positive mothers will shoulder caregiving responsibility (Reyland et al., 2002; Keigher et al., 2005). Kotchick et al. (1997) found that HIV-positive mothers reported poorer mother–child relationship quality and less monitoring of their children than HIV-negative mothers. Forehand et al. (1998) reported more externalising problems and less social competence among children of HIV-positive mothers, while Biggar et al. (2000) found a decrease in academic performance. Children of HIV-positive mothers have also been found to be more withdrawn and to have poorer attention than peers with HIV-negative mothers (Forsyth et al., 1996).

Kotchick et al. (1997) suggest that these effects do not seem to be a function of the mother's ill health; severity of illness was not related to parenting behaviour. A contradictory finding in a study provocatively entitled 'Mother knows best?' (Dorsey et al., 1999) found that mothers reported an increase of child behavioural difficulties through the symptomatic stage of their illness, followed by a decrease in the AIDS stage. In contrast, children reported a steady increase of behavioural difficulties as the illness became more severe. This study is difficult to interpret, because it relied on self-reporting, and because it is unclear whether the mothers or the children were 'correct'. The title of the article makes it clear, however, that the authors think that mothers do not know best – in other words, that they are insufficiently attuned to their children's difficulties.

Other studies, however, suggest different conclusions. Lee and Rotheram-Borus (2001) found that HIV-positive people with more children survived for a longer period of time. This indicates that children serve a protective function. Antle et al. (2001) found that HIV-positive parents cited their children as their primary source of joy. Ingram and Hutchinson (1999) noted that HIV-positive mothers invested more in their parenting role after diagnosis. Black, Nair and Harrington (1994) found that HIV-positive drug-using mothers exhibited more positive attitudes towards and behaviours in parenting than HIV-negative drug-using mothers. Although differences were small, HIV-positive mothers were found to be more tolerant of, involved with and nurturing towards their babies. Unfortunately, non drug-using mothers were not included in the sample. Notably, the title of this article is 'Maternal HIV infection: Parenting and early child development'. The title makes no reference to the fact that all the women in the sample were using drugs, and it was ultimately unclear whether parenting was related to HIV infection or to drug use.

Studies also present mixed conclusions regarding HIV-positive parenting. An article investigating HIV-positive parental fear of contagion (i.e. of infecting their child or being infected by their child), entitled 'Hugs and kisses' (Schuster et al., 2005), found that parents were indeed fearful of contagion, but that this did not have noticeable effects on parent–child interaction. This points to the importance of the distinction between feeling or experience and behaviour, a distinction that is often not made in studies of HIV-positive motherhood. Fear does not always translate into actuality and does not always imply bad parenting. Furthermore, studies on parental deficit do not always sufficiently acknowledge individual variation. A commentary by Stein et al. (2005) seems to introduce contradiction by acknowledging individual variation. The commentary notes that there is limited research on the impact of maternal HIV on children, then goes on to posit a wide range of possible negative consequences for the child of having an HIV-positive mother. This is the focus of the article. It includes, however, the following statement: 'It should be emphasised that despite all the adversity, many women who suffer from HIV-AIDS seem to remain psychologically healthy, cope well, and provide sensitive care and love for their young children' (Stein et al., 2005: 117).

This statement is important, but stands alone and is overwhelmed by the list of possible negative consequences, some of which are conjectured and which are linked to 'compromised parenting and childcare practices' (Stein et al., 2005: 116).

Ingram and Hutchinson (1999), in a rare study that aims to comprehensively address the experiences of HIV-positive mothering, suggest that HIV-positive mothers cope through 'defensive mothering'. The three strategies they outline include preventing the spread of HIV, preparing their children for a motherless future, and protecting themselves through thought control by focusing on their children rather than themselves and through positive reframing. The study defines defensive mothering as a useful and necessary coping mechanism. No link is made to the psychodynamic use of the term. Yet it is clear from the words of the women interviewed that what the authors label 'positive reframing' is a positive reframing, by the authors, of painful emotions dealt with through denial. The concept of defensive mothering thus inadvertently enjoins women to repress their own conflicts and 'avoid succumbing to anxiety and negativity' (Ingram & Hutchinson, 1999: 254). Focus on experiences of motherhood transforms to suggestions for policing identity. It is ironic that a study aimed at addressing the experiences of mothers ultimately only manages to address the way in which mothering is used to help others (children and partners) cope with their experiences.

The principal finding of Black, Nair and Harrington's (1994) study was that HIV-positive drug-using mothers exhibited more positive behaviours and attitudes to parenting than HIV-negative drug-using mothers. They begin their discussion section by adding that HIV-positive mothers appeared to be 'more tolerant and more involved' and 'more nurturant' towards their children (Black, Nair & Harrington, 1994: 608). All their results support this. By the end of their discussion, however, the conclusion emerges that 'many HIV-infected parents do not recognize the emotional needs of their children' (Black, Nair & Harrington, 1994: 612). This statement has no basis in their findings. Their empirical results therefore support positive aspects of HIV-positive (drug-using) mothers, while their inferences regarding HIV-positive mothers (whether drug-using or not) negate these findings and reconstruct the HIV-positive mother as damaging and neglectful. The nurturing mother is replaced by the absent mother; the living mother by the dead mother.

The issue of mother–infant attachment in the context of HIV is particularly loaded, given the extent to which attachment theory has entered into popular parlance. Students are often interested in the impact of maternal HIV on attachment and informal discussion on the subject is common in South Africa. Lectures and textbooks (e.g. Senior, 2002) apply attachment theory to the HIV-positive mother and her infant with the general and untested assumption that attachment will be severely affected. Studies often use HIV as an example, with the assumption accepted that mother–infant attachment will be severely disturbed. For example, Tomlinson, Cooper and Murray (2005) report on a study of attachment in a deprived South African settlement. Challenging another myth about maternal attachment – that poor women in developing countries foster insecure attachments – they found comparable levels of secure attachments in their sample. Relatively high levels of disorganised attachments were found, and it is in relation to this that the example of HIV/AIDS was referred to. They hypothesise that 'the impact of HIV/AIDS as a factor in the preoccupations of women is crucial' (Tomlinson, Cooper & Murray, 2005: 1052). The hypothesis concerning maternal preoccupation is no doubt true, but the statement is used to explain levels of disorganised attachment. Used as an example of the adversity that women face, it can easily be read as a reason for disorganised patterns of attachment.

In fact, attachment issues in the context of HIV are virtually unresearched. One study that directly measured mother–infant attachment (Peterson et al., 2001) concluded, contrary to the authors' expectations, that there was no difference in attachment security between children of HIV-positive and HIV-negative mothers. They found differences in mothers who had AIDS, attributable to AIDS-related ill health. It was not the diagnosis that was associated with poor attachment, but severe illness. This is a distinction that is often not made in studies on HIV-positive motherhood. Furthermore, attachment abnormalities are associated with early mothering. With 70 per cent of mothers surviving for at least the first five years of their children's lives (a statistic that is likely to increase with the increased availability of medication) (Stein et al., 2005), the chances are that most HIV-positive mothers will be asymptomatic during the early attachment-sensitive stage of parenting. This study employed a small sample size and notes the need for more definitive research, but the concept of insecure attachment in the context of HIV seems already to have taken hold.

Finding the HIV-positive mother

A consideration of scientific literature on HIV-positive motherhood demonstrates the narrowness of the range of variables chosen for study, and the sense from the literature of aiming to identify where and how mothers go wrong rather than providing more multifaceted accounts of the experience of being an HIV-positive mother. It should also be noted that the vast majority of these studies are conducted in the global North, while the vast majority of HIV-positive mothers are to be found in the Third

World. Perhaps the thin descriptions found in the literature are an attempt on the part of researchers to avoid succumbing to anxiety and negativity. There is a sense in which these descriptions sanitise the object of 'HIV-positive mother' precisely because of their vagueness. The circumscribed object is less threatening and also less evocative of death and contagion than the object portrayed through the richness of both good and bad. The unidimensional object is easier to comprehend. This may also relate to contemporary constructions of motherhood in which mothers are only of relevance in relation to care of their babies. The HIV-positive mother is simultaneously mother and infectious disease (Patton, 1998), and the thin descriptions found seem to help to keep these two separate.

Within empirical research on HIV-positive mothers lurks either a blankness that leaves the HIV-positive mother unknown and unknowable, or a rupture from which seeps death, guilt and abnormality. The thinness of research findings keeps these ruptures closed by limiting access to the more powerful and painful aspects of the experiences of HIV-positive mothers, while the narrowing down of variables keeps rupture and abnormality under control by keeping aspects of this experience separate and calculable. The threat of the HIV-positive mother is thus diffused. The examples given above of ruptures to composition and rationality suggest that meaning slips and transforms in the act of giving definition to the HIV-positive mother. As soon as the mother is defined as nurturing and living, she is implicitly transformed to being absent and dead. The moment in which she is given definition as a mother is the moment when she is redefined as guilty, withholding and blameworthy. Her active attempts to define herself as normal become the fact of her abnormality.

The themes of death, guilt and abnormality extrapolated from the examples given above are likely to be possible examples of a more general issue regarding the way in which abjection rises unbidden from the study of the HIV-positive mother. The responses arising from these ruptures, it could be argued, are ones of fear and horror that seem to be elicited by the concept of the HIV-positive mother. It is suggested that this may be linked to the coexistence of birth, death and sexuality in the feminine and maternal body responsible for family and children.

Perhaps it is the very difficulty of defining the essence of the HIV-positive mother that prompts the need to define and the impossibility of doing so. Does mother know best? It could be argued that the question, so often implicit in the literature, of whether HIV-positive mothers are good mothers or not is a ridiculous one to pose; obviously, some will be good and some will be bad. Perhaps these examples offer some clues to the challenges faced in researching the experiences of HIV-positive women, and perhaps, too, some clues to the ways in which HIV-positive women are understood by others.

HIV-POSITIVE MOTHERHOOD BETWEEN INNER AND OUTER REALITY

Surrounded as it is by uncertainty and confusion, the process of making meaning of oneself as an HIV-positive mother is explored in this book in terms of how one makes sense of a very impactful inner reality that interacts with the discursive field of outer reality. In this space in between inner and outer reality, the inside and outside of one's body and mind are sites for identity struggle and for making sense of experience. Both psychoanalysis and discourse theory are interested in the interactions between inner and outer reality and in the contingent and shifting nature of these realities. HIV-positive motherhood, located at the collision between HIV and motherhood and between the personal and social, concerns conflict and contradiction, as well as how the profound emotional resonances of motherhood and HIV, together with their discursive meanings, become knotted into subjectivity. It is therefore useful to foreground contradiction, irrationality and the construction of the personal by the social. Because motherhood and HIV are multiple relational, subjectivity is usefully understood in relation to internal and external objects. These suggest some reasons for adopting a theoretical model informed by discourse analysis and psychoanalysis. At the same time, each theoretical influence should not get so carried away in its orthodoxy that it limits itself as a tool for conveying the complexity of HIV-positive motherhood. Psychoanalytic discourse analysis has been critiqued for caricaturing both psychoanalysis and discourse theory, thereby setting up 'good' versus 'bad' theories (Søndergaard, 2002; Wetherell, 1999). Psychoanalysis and post-structuralism articulate with one another, but also limit one another. In pure form, each is purist; but, muddied together, they potentially ask similar questions in different ways. Discourse analysis provides an appropriate tool for exploring processes of construction, meaning making and contradiction on the level of subjectivity in relation to broader social discourses and their participation in power relations. Emphasis on social discourses seems particularly pertinent, given that meanings surrounding HIV/AIDS have fuelled the pandemic. Psychoanalysis provides a tool for understanding both the 'irrational' and the rational, thus valuing processes of fantasy, defence and affect.

Psychoanalytic understandings have not been broadly utilised in understanding HIV. In contrast, HIV research is largely located within the realm of rationality, either through scientific-paradigm research or through research drawing heavily on human rights discourses. The latter is able to open up alternative spaces for the HIV-positive subject, but tends to focus on concepts such as adaptation and coping. Focus on empowerment is liberating, but tends to put a positive spin on human experience. In contrast, a psychoanalytic account would start from the assumption that conflict is inevitable and irrationality the bedrock of experience. This allows conflicts and irrationalities associated with an HIV-positive diagnosis to be examined not as failures, but as inevitable in the face of painful knowledge. In its own way, this is potentially liberating in its ability to simply acknowledge that this kind of experience is one of both internal struggle and struggle against broader social discourses. There is also limited employment of psychodynamic concepts in understanding the social aspects of the pandemic. Many social and psychological analyses of HIV/AIDS, however, describe processes that can be clearly linked to issues of irrationality, but are seldom framed as such. The silence so often described in relation to HIV has links to denial; prejudice can be clearly linked to processes of splitting and projection. That HIV/AIDS intersects so strongly with issues of sexuality, life and death, as well as with fear, hope, love and hate, further suggests the applicability of a psychoanalytic framework.

Psychoanalysis offers a process for understanding interview material, suggesting a way of listening for multiple levels of meaning. It is particularly useful in its recognition of the unspeakable and the unbearable, and also offers a framework for tolerance of the painful terrain of HIV-positive motherhood. Given the nebulous and socially produced nature of HIV-positive motherhood, psychoanalysis proposes fruitful understandings of both the centrality of fantasy and of fear and desire in the struggle to make sense of life. Psychoanalysis has also developed sophisticated ways of understanding the workings of affect, e.g. guilt, anger, envy and anxiety, central to interview material. It offers ways of understanding meaning proliferating out of control, as well as hearing the unsaid and the silenced.

'Psychoanalysis' is deliberately employed here as a methodological tool, and not as a particular theory. This is partly because there is a divergence of different theories under the psychoanalytic umbrella, and many of these theories have been critiqued for their Western and bourgeois bias (Frosh, 1997a). Preference for process issues such as fantasy, affect and defence does not require strict adherence to a particular psychoanalytic school, and thus helps to limit the risk of imposing grand theory on the narratives of HIV-positive mothers. The contradictory and split nature of HIV-positive motherhood, as well as the extent to which the HIV-positive mother becomes a recipient of projections, lends itself to a Kleinian approach, while Winnicott has been useful because of the centrality of motherhood to his theory and in his understanding of experience. Winnicott (1971) understands experience as the thing that happens in between inner and outer reality, in a transitional or potential space out of which flows the search for the self. Thinking about HIV-positive maternal experience in this way highlights the transitional sense of becoming a mother and becoming HIV-positive, rather than simply evoking a category with simple descriptors that match the dual diagnosis.

It also emphasises the interaction, rather than opposition, between inner and outer experience. Winnicott's understanding of experience is largely personal and individual, but he does recognise the location of cultural experience between inner and outer reality and in 'the potential space between the individual and the environment' (Winnicott, 1971: 103). The environment is introjected into the individual and inner reality is projected onto the environment. This is similar to Klein's understanding of the ways in which the external enters the internal world, and vice versa, although Klein's conception is arguably much more interactive (e.g. see Klein, 1940). It then becomes possible to wonder about the ways in which discourses (e.g. of being HIV-positive or of motherhood) may enter inner reality and the ways in which discursively constructed objects offer opportunities for projection. HIV-positive motherhood, then, is an experience in the sense that it is deeply personal and always bound up in discourse.

Discourses are systems of meanings and metaphors that construct particular subjects and objects within a set of power relations (Foucault, 1971; Parker, 1992). Discourses of race or gender, for example, tell particular stories about particular kinds of people. These stories are socially and historically specific. They also construct particular kinds of bodies and particular kinds of identities. Similarly, discourses of motherhood and discourses of HIV offer 'social constructs [that] 'fix' the range of identity positions available to people' (Frosh, Phoenix & Pattman, 2003: 39). Contradictory discourses offer different subject positions. Taking up a subject position means being positioned in relation to the system of meanings offered by a particular discourse (Davies & Harré, 1990). Being positioned in relation to discourse also implies being positioned within the power relations associated with that discourse, requiring strategies of self-surveillance or policing. In this way, one is subjected to and the subject of a particular discourse (Foucault, 1975; Rose, 1989).

Weedon's definition of discourse, with its inclusion of the unconscious and the equal importance of body and mind, has been useful:

Discourses ... are ways of constituting knowledge, together with the social practices, forms of subjectivity and power relations which inhere in such knowledges and the relations between them. Discourses are more than ways of thinking and producing meaning. They constitute the 'nature' of the body, unconscious and conscious mind and emotional life of the subjects they seek to govern. Neither the body nor thoughts and feelings have meaning outside their discursive articulation, but the ways in which discourse constitutes the minds and bodies of individuals is always part of a wider network of power relations, often with institutional bases (Weedon, 1987 in Davies, 1990: 505).

The social subject is therefore positioned within discourse in both unconscious and conscious ways and constructed through body and mind. The inclusion of mind and body into understandings of discourse is important in the context of HIV-positive motherhood.

It has been argued that the inclusion of discourse analysis into psycho analysis potentially avoids the psychoanalytic pitfalls of individualising, pathologising and universalising (Elliott & Frosh, 1995). Conversely, discourse analysis is aided by the complexity of psychoanalytic accounts (Flax, 1993), and this allows one to answer the question of *why* subjects invest in particular subject positions (Frosh, Phoenix & Pattman, 2000) and how such emotional investments take place (Hollway, 1989; Hollway & Jefferson, 2000). The two theories have also become increasingly influenced by one another (Billig, 1999; Elliott & Spezzano, 2000). However, much discussion, in psychology at least, has been primarily theoretical and methodological, with actual application considered secondary (Howarth, 2003). Both psychoanalysis (Parker, 2003; Wetherell, 1999) and post-modernism (Elliott & Spezzano, 2000) have been critiqued for imposing meta-narratives onto their subjects, rendering neither value free. Important limits need to be placed upon these endeavours. Both discourse analysis and psychoanalysis rely heavily on interpretation, and such interpretations need to be made respectfully and cautiously (Frosh, Phoenix

& Pattman, 2003). Psychoanalytic discourse analysis has been critiqued for assuming the existence of a hidden reality that only those in the know can uncover (Wetherell, 1999). Hollway and Jefferson (2000) have been critiqued for using 'psychoanalysis as a form of truth' (Parker, 2003: 313) and for individualising and psychologising research participants in a mystical search for unconscious motivation (Wetherell, 2005). Walkerdine, Lucey and Melody (2001) could similarly be critiqued for relying on concepts of transference and counter-transference that are no doubt present in a research interview, but are elusive enough within psychotherapy and therefore difficult to interpret in a research interview.

Two points need to be made in regard to this book. Firstly, a research interview is very different from ongoing psychotherapy. Even when more than one interview is conducted, the expectations of both parties are different and the relationship is not sufficiently established for the unconscious to be accessed or transference to be properly understood. Secondly, psychoanalytic discourse analysis usually asks questions about the psychodynamic inflections of broader social identities. Research questions do not concern the psychodynamics of an individual (which the first point suggests are elusive anyway). Despite this, there is a tendency in such work to analyse individuals (including their unconscious motivations) in order to answer questions about groups.

Recognising that the distinction between the individual and the group is spurious, it is suggested that questions regarding the interaction between personal and social identities themselves need to blur the boundaries between self and others. The method employed here aims to maintain the tension between meanings elicited through an individual's story and the relationships of these meanings to the stories and subject positions of others. Individual stories are therefore read through the stories of others so that the question of why a particular woman positions herself in a particular way is answered through both her own account and the accounts of others. Holding this tension also involves recognising that the aim is not to uncover individual unconscious motivations, which risks pathologising individuals. Rather, it is to examine relationships among meanings in order to suggest some of the conflicts and tensions involved in HIV-positive motherhood – to look for the ways in which the unsaid or the 'eccentric, the erratic and the excessive' (Frosh, 2002: 123) promote understanding of the multiplicities and contradictions within and between subject positions in this study. Nothing can be definitively said about an individual's unconscious.

Perhaps the most productive similarity between the two theories concerns their conception of subjectivity, which is of importance to this book. It has been suggested that both theories challenge rationalist notions of personhood, suggesting that identity is non-unitary, multiple, fragmented and contradictory (Henriques et al., 1984; Wetherell, 2002). In both cases, the subject can be seen as constructed and reconstructed, either by language and discursive history or by processes of reconstructing the self through relationship histories (Henriques et. al., 1984).

The emphasis on irrationality, by psychoanalysis on the unconscious and by discourse theory on the incorporation of arbitrary systems of knowledge and power, links to the suspicion of both theories regarding the objectivity of 'truth'. This introduces suspicion of moral discourses regarding motherhood and HIV, while highlighting that fantasy is not separate from 'truth', and that public and private fantasies exist in dynamic relation to one another (Frosh, 1997b).

Contradiction and conflict are central. In discourse theory, subjectivity is contradictory, because of the subject's positioning in multiple discourses. The psychoanalytic concept of conflict evokes a similar sense of a subject caught between multiple imperatives, although this process is seen as more affect laden and irrational. Both senses are important in relation to HIV-positive motherhood, in which discursive contradiction and psychodynamic conflict are potentially mutually related.

The incorporation of the body into the study of subjectivity is imperative to this research, since both motherhood and HIV are bodily experiences, with psychodynamic and discursive meanings attached to these bodies.

For discourse theory, bodies under surveillance foster a process of self-surveillance (Foucault, 1975; Rose, 1989) and discourse inscribes the body in particular ways (Butler, 1993). Psychoanalysis recognises the centrality of the body in the making of identity, as well as the constitutive nature of the experience of one's body.

Further, both HIV and motherhood involve complex losses of identity. Frosh, Phoenix and Pattman (2000; 2003), following Butler (1990; 1997), have proposed that psychoanalytic discourse analysis is able to explore the losses associated with entering into gendered subject positions. They argue that entering into gendered identities is necessarily a process of repudiation, and that taking up particular identities produces discursive contradictions and defensive subject positions marked by anxiety, loss and sadness. This has been an influential framework not only in relation to identity losses on entering HIV-positive or maternal identities, but also in relation to broader losses implied by the issues of sexuality, life and death evoked through the simultaneous experience of motherhood and HIV. Both approaches, therefore, provide theoretical and methodological frameworks, and both are able to explore both process and content.

The constructed and multiple subject inserted into fantasies of truth in contradictory and conflictual ways is also not an individual entity. Both theories emphasise the blurring of boundaries between self and other (Elliott & Frosh, 1995). Comprehending oneself as HIV-positive or as a mother has to be done relationally, and is potentially a process by which one becomes what another imagines one to be. This process is understood as imbued with productive power: discursive and psychodynamic meanings produce subjectivity. For Foucault (1975), power resides in discourse; power/knowledge combinations produce subject positions. In other words, power produces the desire to monitor oneself into a particular discursive identity (Rose, 1989; 1998). In the psychoanalytic account, one's identity is produced through power, desire and loss. The power of discourse and the power of desire and repudiation are both understood as productive. Power produces subjectivity discursively within systems of ideas and meanings, and psychodynamically through relationship and affect. Both motherhood and HIV produce certain kinds of power relations, which, it will be suggested, are simultaneously personal and social.

Power, in the discursive account, produces subjectivity through the operations of difference, or the construction of binary oppositions that make discourse a fundamentally comparative process. Discourse theory is often interested in political binaries, such as gender, race or sexuality, and in deconstructing these differences for political purposes. Psychoanalysis is also seen as potentially politically useful in understanding these binaries as irrational and artificial:

> What is suggested by both psychoanalysis and postmodernism is that imagined worlds of this kind work by smoothing out the rough edges, homogenising what should be heterogeneous, making monolithic what should be plural, and, in their purity, killing off all the rest (Frosh, 2002: 133).

Black HIV-positive mothers occupy at least a triple position in which they are on the 'different' side of the binary (black; HIV-positive; mothers). If power and difference are fuelled by fantasy, it is unsurprising that this conglomeration of subject positions produces such powerful discourses. Discourses do not just construct difference, but seem to be particularly fascinated by difference. Fascination and imagination proliferate discourse as much as do power relations.

These themes are implicit in the chapters to come. The book should not be read as a diagnosis of HIV-positive motherhood, since this category itself is a fantasy of homogeneity. Its intention is to explore the meanings and experiences of HIV-positive motherhood, foregrounding the stories that HIV-positive mothers told and their existence between inner and outer reality. The following chapters therefore explore constructions and fantasies of HIV-positive motherhood from the perspective of real mothers.

5. Minding Baby's Body

One would expect this chapter, which begins a closer analysis of HIV-positive motherhood, to be about mothers and not about babies. Contemplating the body and mind of the HIV-positive mother, however, inevitably involves the mother contemplating her baby. Imagining a sick and dying baby invokes something quite different from imagining a sick and dying adult, for the onlooker as well as for the mother herself. The question implied is not 'What has this baby *done* to deserve this?' but the more rhetorical 'What has this baby done to *deserve* this?' The innocence of babies and the pathos elicited by something so small and new becoming sick means that the baby's body, so close to the body of the mother, comes more easily into focus. This is magnified by social expectations that the mother's body be utterly secondary to the baby's body and the mother's mind selflessly turned away from itself. When the mother is HIV-positive, with the potential that the baby might be too, HIV insinuates itself into the eclipse. Looking at one's own HIV-positive body entails looking at an infected body; looking as a mother, this body is primarily – if only potentially – infecting.

The potentiality of infection preoccupied experiences of motherhood in this study. Mothers potentially infect their babies during pregnancy or, more likely, during labour. The probability of infection is 31 per cent, reduced by a single dose of Nevirapine to 13 per cent (Department of Health, 2002). This means that the majority of children born to HIV-positive mothers are negative (Sherr, 1999). Because of the stigma associated with the disease, mother-to-child-transmission is taken much more seriously than other transmissible diseases with equivalent or higher transmission rates. After birth, mothers can only infect their babies through breastfeeding, and even then there is only an 8 per cent probability of infection.

Imagining sick and dying babies, then, is the most frightening, but not the most likely outcome. Preoccupation with infection reflects potentiality and not probability, and this preoccupation is no doubt associated with prejudice, particularly regarding the infectious potential of mothers. Another reason, however, why constructions of motherhood were dominated by concerns of infection is likely to be related to the uncertainty that mothers endure before they know whether their babies are infected or not. Since babies cannot be immediately tested, their HIV status is initially unknown. This means that women become mothers to babies and mother them without knowing the implications of their own infection for their babies' future. This uncertainty easily trumps probability.

This chapter, perhaps unsurprisingly then, is hardly about the mother at all – but it is also about nothing else. If the HIV-positive body was relatively ungendered, asexual and non-procreative – not a mother's body – then the baby's body is primarily in the mind of the mother minding (and minding about) the baby's body. The process of monitoring and caring for the baby's body (invoking the baby as well as the mother) is visceral and incites an unarticulable quality of anxiety in motherhood. Discourse fails in the construction of subjectivity as questions about the baby float free and are silent, and HIV occupies a position in between mother and baby.

MINDING BABY'S BODY: 'OH GOD, MAYBE HE'S LIKE ME'

Monitoring one's own HIV-positive body entails a process of observing the boundaries of the body: at what point will the invisible inside become visible outside? How will what goes into the body (both materially and symbolically) interact with the virus already there, and how can what is inside be kept on the boundaries of identity and be prevented from erupting on one's surface, for all to see? Monitoring one's baby's body entails a somewhat different process in at least four ways. Firstly, the invisible inside the baby's body is a mystery until the mother knows the baby's disease status. Searching the baby's body is a process not of searching for signs of an infection already there, but one of knowing that this body has the potential to be infected, of trying to guess what is under the surface.

Secondly, there is a certainty within this uncertainty: if the baby is HIV infected, this time bomb inside was planted by the mother. Parents are often delighted when others see physical similarities between them and their children. 'My child looks like me' is proof of connection and a point of identification: 'My child is like me.' HIV-positive mothers often described constantly scanning the baby's body, searching for clues that the baby is either safe from infection or is not: that the baby is, or is not, like the mother. Zodwa captures the horror of this uncertainty, which, if realised, confirms the certainty that the mother has turned the baby into herself: 'not knowing how he is, it's gonna make me feel like, "Oh God, maybe he's like me".'

Thirdly, the possibility of this identification cannot be separated from the innocence of babies, and therefore cannot be separated from the dread that the mother is responsible for doing this to the baby. The bodies of babies are small and unmarked by experience. Nonyameko captures this unelaborable combination of innocence and dread:

I said, 'me, I can be positive; I don't, it's okay'. But only for this young baby, the poor little baby, to come out positive, it's really unfair, you know that .... Just for the baby, for the sake of the baby. She didn't know anything. You know.

The horror of one's own body pales in comparison to the horror of the infection of innocence. The dread of identification – of similarity – also evokes the fundamental difference of the greater importance of the baby's body and of what was often framed as the baby's greater claim to sympathy, help and care.

Fourthly, while there are things to do and doctors to consult in relation to the mother's body where infection is known, the uncertainty of not knowing the baby's status means that one does not know what kind of sympathy, help and care the baby needs. There is a certain paralysis in having to wait, to endure the period of not knowing, but constantly trying to guess what one may have done to one's baby. While still pregnant, Charity imagines this period of not knowing her baby's status:

> *Charity:* It will be difficult for me. But as long as the baby is quite fine, then *ja.* I want the baby to be fine. Has to come out fine.
> *CL:* What, what will it mean for you if she wasn't fine?
> *Charity:* There's nothing I can do, but .... [pause]
> *CL:* How would you feel?
> *Charity:* Mm, I don't know [laughs], I can't even know.
> *CL:* You don't even want to think about it?
> *Charity:* Yes. It's an innocent child.

Charity's insistence that the baby 'has to come out fine' is plagued by the possibility that this will not happen and by her helplessness in being able to do 'nothing'. In this extract, she keeps losing words, finding herself lacking in knowledge and confronted with the innocence of her child. Across interviews, there was a sense of women holding their breaths through this uncertainty, not quite being able to say one way or another and consequently not quite being able to speak.

These four differences between the mother and the baby are crucial, and tinge the mother's care of her baby's body with uncertainty and dread. In the analysis presented below, each difference is intertwined with meanings of motherhood contemplated through trying to find meaning in the baby's body. The baby's body becomes the object of recursive searching and imagination, and the promise of medicine to protect the baby's body cannot quite contain meaning and uncertainty about the baby's HIV status and maintains meaning in a state of flux.

IMAGINING THE BABY'S BODY

A notable difference between interviews with pregnant women and those who had given birth concerned discussion in which women imagined their baby's bodies. This coincides with a central difference between pregnancy and motherhood: in the former, the baby is inside the mother's body and cannot be seen. If the baby can be seen, even if HIV cannot, there is a body to search. If the baby is hidden, one has only one's imagination. Perhaps this is why Charity, heavily pregnant, repeatedly said that all she wanted was to 'see' her baby. Without any visual proof, she could not begin to evaluate whether her baby was HIV-positive or -negative. When her baby was born, she wanted to do an interview as soon as she could so that I could see that her baby looked healthy.

Having to rely on imagination, one might expect that pregnant women alternately imagined either perfect children or had frightening fantasies of their babies' bodies. This would be consistent with the experiences of 'normal' mothers, who often fantasise as well as dream frightening and vivid scenes of horror. Raphael-Leff (1997) suggests that dreams and fantasies usually accelerate during pregnancy to the point that practitioners unaware of the normality of this process are likely to think that their patients are psychotic. Pregnant women, when interviewed, however, fantasised and dreamed very little about their babies, and overwhelmingly imagined good things. When asked to imagine their babies, women often responded with the same sense of finality with which Charity contemplated her child's status above (it 'has to come out fine'). They imagined the bodies of their babies as boys or girls, imagined very little about what kind of personality the baby would have other than 'happy' and had little to say about what their babies would look like. Underlying these responses, however, was often an insistence, as in Charity's extract above, that their babies were 'healthy'. Amara simply says that she imagines 'a healthy baby. Just a nice happy baby'. She allows no opportunity for any other alternatives. Thandiwe imagines her baby as a girl,

> and then I'm very happy and I'm seeing a child, it's a clever child, because I can just hear her kicking on my stomach, playing. I see all those things, *ja*. So I'm very pleased and I'm seeing her as a healthy baby, mm. A baby that has got a future, *ja*. So I'm very positive about her, *ja*.

Thandiwe imagines a 'clever' girl and she is filled with joy. Essential to her joy as a mother is not only that her baby is clever, but that she is 'healthy' and has a future. Thandiwe is making a veiled reference to the possibility of HIV, which would deprive her child of health and a future, but her certainty that her child is healthy combats this threat. HIV is present in her comment, but only by implication and negation.

When her baby is born, however, Thandiwe is racked with uncertainty and desperately searches her baby's body for clues about her baby's status. When her baby cannot be seen, certainty and optimism can be maintained, but as soon as her baby's body is visible – and looks healthy – she can no longer defend herself against her guilt and fear that she has infected her baby. Charity's certainty during pregnancy was answered with great relief when she was finally able to see her baby and experience the joy of her health, but this too introduced uncertainty and the ruthless search for signs of either health or infection.

The correspondence between certainty in the unseen and uncertainty once the baby's body can be seen, however, is easily reversed. Neo, for example, had 'seen' her baby on a scan when pregnant. She looks back to the time before she had an image of her baby's body and remembers imagining fearful things:

> *Neo: Ja*, you know, you just dream of your child being positive – not healthy. That hair loss, whatever. So you always think about those things, you know, *ja*, that makes you very sad, mm …. You just imagine a monster, you know, [laughs] coming out from you. But now that I went for a sonar and I did a 3-D scan, you know, so I, I was able to watch him, that's all.
>
> *CL:* Okay.
>
> *Neo:* But very much happy, you know, mm.
>
> *CL:* And that helps?
>
> *Neo: Ja*, it helped a lot, because you could see that he's healthy and fine, you know.

In retrospect, Neo refers to a monster fantasy common to many pregnant women, but here related exclusively to HIV. Being able to see her baby gave Neo some reassurance that 'he's healthy and fine'. When more frightening fantasies were mentioned by women, this was often done in retrospect. If the fantasy has passed (or can be said to have passed), it is less frightening. Amara took part in three interviews during pregnancy, in which she maintained that she never dreamed about her baby and only imagined good in her baby's body. After her baby was born, she expressed relief. It was only at this point that she could say how frightened she had been:

> Hey, yoh, yoh, I was so worried, you know, there were so many things in my mind, so confused, and if the baby is not alive – what if the baby is nearly disabled or something is wrong, you know. I was so worried. Because I could see now that the baby now is about to be born, so I don't know what kind of a baby, *ja*. I was so worried, but I was just looking forward to that baby. I was worried *'cos* I didn't know, you know.

During pregnancy, Amara would not allow space for what she 'didn't know'. Looking back from the safety of relief, she expresses the extent of her worry.

The descriptions given by Neo and Amara illustrate the power of the fantasies that did emerge in relation to the baby's body, as well as their interrelatedness with HIV. When women did report dreams, they were often frighteningly graphic, involving mangled bodies, often taking place in hospital and always related to HIV. Joyce expresses the exclusivity of HIV in her dreams. After describing a dream in which a nurse takes her baby away from her after delivery and returns to say that the baby is dead, she reflects on what the dream might mean: 'It's this HIV thing. This thing that I think. Otherwise some other things I don't worry about. It's just this HIV.' Joyce does not have anxieties for her baby extrinsic to HIV. The threat of infection eclipses all the other fantasies that many women have about their babies. The relative absence of dreams and fantasies suggests their danger in relation to the omnipresence of HIV, and another way in which women monitored their own minds, this time as mothers, in order to keep infection in place.

OBSERVING THE BABY'S BODY

Once the baby is born and the mother is in daily intimate contact with her baby's body, the search for and containment of infection becomes considerably more direct. This is complicated by not knowing the baby's HIV status and by the impossibility of trying to guess it. Babies are generally vulnerable to infection and are likely to become sick. The dilemma lies in how to interpret sickness, or, for that matter, health. Because the disease is unpredictable, it is possible that a healthy baby is HIV-positive and a sick baby HIV-negative. Any sign of health or illness could therefore be interpreted either way.

Within these impossibilities, the compulsion to constantly examine the baby's body for signs of infection was amplified rather than diminished. Descriptions abounded of careful observation of the baby – a common process in early motherhood, through which women anxiously search their babies' bodies in case something is wrong, but here almost strictly reserved for monitoring the possibility of HIV infection. Kuli, for example, describes 'observance' as the most important aspect of motherhood. The word implies both observation of baby and observance of a ritual. Carefully monitoring her baby helps her to answer the burning question of her baby's status. At different points in her interview, however, she finds contradictory answers. At one point, observing her baby leads her to find hope that her baby is 'normal': 'When I talk to her, she's already normal, recognised my voice and she always look me inside my eyes and it shows that she, she's starting, she's teaching me herself to be normal.'

This comment refers to her worries about her baby's health. Here, she categorises her baby as 'normal'. Her duty as a mother is to allow her baby to teach her to be normal in return, and not to be hypervigilant of her baby. At another point, however, 'observance' means categorising her baby as 'special'. She explains: 'She's not like other children, *ja*, she needs special care, *ja*. I think she needs the special care; I should observe her, time, eh, day by day, *ja*. To see if there's some changes, rashes, eh, thrush, whatever.'

Although Kuli does not know her baby's status, she feels obliged to place her in a separate category to 'other children' because of the risk that she might be infected. She does not know if her daughter belongs in this category, but she is not prepared to take chances. She describes a minute procedure of observation, and her vigilance has a defined target: her baby's health. She must notice the slightest change to her baby's body. Implicit in her metaphor of 'changes' is the implication of progression. Many babies get rashes or thrush, but will this progress into HIV? To be a good mother, Kuli needs to accomplish the impossible task of seeing through her baby's body to the secrets it holds within and which she cannot yet know.

This double invisibility, the as-yet-unseen potential of the existence of an invisible virus, often played into the monitoring of the baby's body and the uncertainty of knowing one's baby's status. Within this uncertainty, the guessing can go both ways. Mandisa, for example, describes her fantasies when observing her baby's sick body. She acknowledges that her uncertainty, while terrible, allows some relief, because she does not have a confirmed positive diagnosis. 'Not knowing' holds the possibility that her child may be negative.

> Not knowing is very terrible, it's very terrible, but it brings some relief as well, because with knowing I think I'm gonna have that thing of saying, 'Is he gonna be fine?' But not knowing as well, it's frustrating. Because whenever he's sick, I feel that it has something to do with it, even when he's got a cold. The last time he was very sick, he had this terrible cold and I thought maybe he's too sick and then I took him to the hospital and they told me it was just some bronchitis – flu or something like that – but it was horrible.

Significantly, 'not knowing' implicitly presumes that 'knowing' will mean knowing that her baby is positive: 'knowing' means facing the question 'Is he gonna be fine?' when he gets sick. She immediately turns to the flipside of the equation: that 'not knowing' allows the possibility that he may be HIV-positive – that 'it' is responsible when he is sick – describing the oft-repeated process of searching for signs of infection. If she knows, it means she knows that he is positive. If she does not yet know, it means she does not yet know that he is positive. Either alternative leads to infection. In the moment of acknowledging the 'relief' in knowing nothing other than that he might be negative, infection thwarts her.

Trying to guess the status of the invisible inside also involves a search for signs on the body. A few minutes later, Mandisa describes the flipside of looking – looking not for signs of infection, but for signs of health. I ask her whether she tries to guess whether he is positive or negative:

> I always do that, you know, and it's because of the way he is; I have this thing of he's negative. When you look at him, he's very active, you know, and he's growing well. So I have this thing, I have this thing where I say, 'No, he couldn't be positive'. Because of the way he is.

Mandisa here looks at her baby and tries to evaluate his health. Echoing a typical argument, she sees that he is growing well and is active and the proof in this moment that he is negative is stronger than the proof that he is positive when he is sick.

Observing the baby's body is accomplished in a terrain of opposites and reversals. Kuli requires herself to look for normality and specialness and to help her baby by seeing health as well as seeing sickness. Each is accomplished separately, and the contradiction is unacknowledged. Mandisa similarly looks at her baby and finds proof of both sickness and health, and in the moment of finding either, refutes the possibility of the other. Any point of knowledge can be undone in a moment. The process of observance is also one of training a medical eye on one's baby in an attempt to diagnose. If one can correctly read the signs, perhaps uncertainty can be overcome. This, too, is an impossible task and one that the medical establishment also promises, but fails, to achieve.

THE PROMISE OF MEDICINE

Women often stressed the importance of going to the doctor and being proactive in protecting their own bodies. They similarly described the importance of seeking medical attention for their babies. Dikeledi stresses the urgency of medical intervention if there is anything wrong with her baby, no matter how small:

> What if the virus is coming out, and then the baby and everything? So, like, I will, get up and run to the doctor, do this, do this, yo, I won't sleep, I will just hold him with my hands, like, you know ... [pause] whenever I think about. So if, for instance, if maybe I wasn't told that I was positive, like if he was sick, I would just take it as a normal thing.

Dikeledi recognises that her baby can be sick and it may just be a 'normal thing', but her knowledge of her own status prompts a desperate need to 'get up and run'. She describes an incident where a doctor said that her baby's diarrhoea was normal, 'so the doctor just said, he said, "you are mad. You are mad". ... But I felt that, you know, it was better to come than not to come.' The doctor thinks she is being over-zealous, but this is far less important to her than her need to be careful in case the diarrhoea is not normal.

Where medical discourse was constructed as a means of salvation (albeit contradictory) in relation to one's own body, it faltered more explicitly in relation to one's baby. Ayanda describes the desperate imperative to seek treatment by comparing her experience of her baby to that of her older child, born years before Ayanda was diagnosed:

> Even sometimes the baby, this one if he gets diarrhoea, I must run! I know I must make some water for him, but I don't want to rely on that water too much. If it's more than three days, I must make sure there's some, get some treatment. Even, every, everything that he does, I must make sure it's perfect, you know. You know, you get some treatment very soon. That one [referring to her first child, eight years old at the time], I could cope and I'd say, 'haai, it'll be fine. It's just colds, he's going to be fine. I'll buy some medicine.' But with this one, it's different, because I know his status.

At this point, Ayanda does not in fact 'know his status'; all she knows is the possibility of him being positive and the urgency this provokes. The doctor's authority, however, does not stem her desperation. She describes her last visit to her son's doctor:

> The baby, you check the baby, you look everywhere; it's very hard. These are hard times, you know, you look, even if you see this, like now I told the doctor that this rash, he says to me, 'haai, this rash is normal'. I said, 'please give me something'. He just gave me the aqueous cream [laughs]. But he said it's normal, but I don't want to see anything nasty, you know, anything you think is not normal to me.

Ayanda captures her hypervigilance regarding her baby's body. She laughs wryly at herself for failing to be consoled by medical opinion, for worrying more than the doctor thinks is warranted. Medical discourse fails here, not because of its inability to adequately treat, but because there is an excess that medicine cannot take away. Even if the doctor correctly diagnoses and treats the rash, this is not powerful enough to eradicate the threat of her baby's infection; Ayanda does not want 'to see anything nasty'. The rash may be medically normal to the doctor, but for Ayanda this is meaningless, because it is not normal to her. Perhaps it is not a sign of infection (but, of course, perhaps it is). It is, however, a sign that her baby might be like her and is therefore a reminder of her baby's potential.

Amara similarly describes the centrality of medicine and its ultimate failure. In one interview, she discusses a car accident that she and her baby were involved in. This event does not lead her to worry about her own HIV status, but the threat of the accident to her baby immediately evokes her baby's possible status. She worries that if her baby is positive, an accident would be detrimental, and immediately seeks medical intervention. One medical opinion, however, does not suffice:

> *Ja*, the baby's okay, I took him to three doctors yesterday, because I was so scared that the hospital, because they took us to hospital, then they said, 'no the baby's fine'. Then yesterday I said, 'uh-uh, I can't sit, because maybe she's fine, but maybe there's something they missed', so I took her to the doctor; the first doctor said she's okay, [then] the other doctor, and then I just said, 'okay, that means she's fine'.

Even when Amara procures three medical opinions, she is only temporarily appeased. Later in the interview she again questions whether she can rely on the doctors' diagnoses: 'So I must take her back tomorrow, back here, so he can check again. I must bring her again, just to make sure.' It seems that no amount of checking is enough; nothing can quite satisfy her that her daughter is safe. Perhaps the accident does not evoke her own HIV status because she knows that the invisible virus is present. In the case of her baby, HIV immediately springs to mind, because she can only guess what is under the surface of the body.

Although the medical establishment cannot initially provide a definitive answer, it does provide Nevirapine, and thereby the promise that the baby is more likely to be safe. Being able to take Nevirapine was important to the mothers, because it offered hope and allowed them to feel proactive in the protection of their babies. The fact of Nevirapine was often called upon when women observed their babies, either to reassure them that an illness was not HIV related or to confirm observations of health. Dikeledi, who knows that her baby is negative, looks for health in her baby, and finds this with the help of her knowledge that Nevirapine worked to save her baby. Even within this certainty of his status, however, she describes a process of searching, of not being entirely sure that what she knows is true:

> And he's a fresh baby; he eats a lot you know. *Ja*. Whenever I even look at him, I just say, 'ah God, maybe they lied about the test', but look at my son; they didn't lie. The Nevirapine is the one which filled that. It did work.

Faced with a negative diagnosis and a healthy body, Dikeledi worries that 'they lied'. It is not clear whether she is wondering whether they lied about her positive status or about her baby's negative status (i.e. whether her baby is or is not like her). Her confusion is settled because Nevirapine can be relied upon – this is what allows her to believe that he is healthy.

The drug, then, offers one possibility of resistance against uncertainty, but even this does not eradicate the anxiety of infection and of the 'Oh God, maybe he's like me' response. Neither does it entirely ease the trauma of having to wait for the baby's result. Hlengiwe was 'excited that, hey, my baby got this Nevirapine', but when she discovered how long she would have to wait to know whether Nevirapine 'worked', she began to distrust her excitement. She felt that Nevirapine could give her a dangerously false sense of hope:

> Because you've been waiting and waiting until that result that, no, my baby is fine and trying to do your best for the little one, but at the end of the day, all that effort, it's gone to waste, because at the end of the day, the baby's going to die before you die. Because a baby cannot fight for himself, you have to help him fight, but at the end of the day, he's going to die. Yes.

Hlengiwe cannot trust her excitement that her baby has access to Nevirapine, because she knows that its success is not guaranteed. Even the most concrete of medical interventions cannot resolve the fear of the worst – that her baby may die and that her care has 'gone to waste'. Nevirapine cannot stop the possibility of her own failure as a mother – that she failed to 'help him fight'.

For Thandiwe, this failure to provide a guarantee is linked to the impossibility of knowing whether or not she has found signs of HIV on her baby's body. She cannot decide whether her baby looks healthy or sick and cannot decide what either predicts, because sometimes HIV-positive babies 'look normal; sometimes others, they do die quick, you know'. This double uncertainty about whether her baby looks healthy or not and about whether healthy babies are positive and sick ones negative or vice versa leads her to worry about whether Nevirapine actually works. In the face of the impossibility of predicting HIV status from one's baby's body, Nevirapine loses its predictive power as well.

Lukanyo similarly expresses her confusion about how to make sense of her baby's body and also about the hope medicine may offer. She is wrestling with the dilemma that healthy babies can be sick and sick babies healthy:

> Mm, I'm not sure because of, like, the doctor was, they told me last, you know, they said the baby can look very good, *né*, and fat, but he can still be sick. So, ah, it's something that I, I don't want to think about it too much …. Like, before I used to, to say he's positive, *né*?

Because he was having glands, *né?* When he was born, he was having glands here and on the armpits; he still has those ones, *né,* but the other doctors they told me that those glands, there can be some infections, not that he's sick. So even myself, sometimes I become confused, *né?* ... I don't know really which is which.

Medical opinion tells her that healthy babies can be HIV-positive ('can still be sick') and at another point tells her that her baby's swollen glands could mean nothing ('not that he's sick'). This is the reality of the disease, but it leaves her in confusion and reticent about investing in the hope of medical opinion. Medicine warns her not to be complacent, but also reassures her; she is left with no place to stand in relation to her baby. She comments in a subsequent interview that doctors have said her baby is probably not HIV-positive, 'because if he has AIDS, he'll become soft'. She has, however, seen healthy-looking babies diagnosed HIV-positive, 'so it's just difficult to see it'. She tries to reassure herself, but fails on the basis of the invisibility of the disease, of the impossibility of looking and seeing. Medical opinion cannot help, because Lukanyo cannot allow herself to become complacent; the baby's body cannot be contained by medical discourse, because those little glands or that activity she sees cannot contain the fear that she has infected her baby. The promise of medicine fails, because it cannot take away the uncertainty.

THE END OF THE WAIT

If medical opinion is not powerful enough in the face of the possibility of HIV, medical science can at least eventually supply a definitive answer to the question of infection when the baby is old enough to be tested. Some of the women interviewed did not yet know their babies' status. Of those who did, only two women with HIV-positive babies were interviewed. This is no doubt partly because Nevirapine reduced the probability of transmitting to the baby and partly because of the shame attached to having an HIV-positive baby. Both women whose babies were diagnosed positive, while devastated, expressed some relief that the period of uncertainty was over. This was also the overwhelming response from women whose babies were negative. The diagnosis provided respite from the paralysis of waiting and allowed mothers to exhale. Women consistently described their relief that their babies were negative. They no longer had to worry about whether their babies would become sick and die from AIDS, and this allowed them to feel that their babies were safe. They also no longer needed to feel guilty about being infecting mothers, and the relief this brought was immense. Women described being able to relax in their caring for their babies and being able to shift HIV out of centre stage in the mother–infant relationship. Women also described experiencing a new lease on life themselves. Mandisa, who sent a text message to tell me her news, wrote, 'I have never felt better in my life. My son is negative and this motivates me. Carol, I wish you were here when they gave me the results'.

Mandisa describes a highlight in her life where she feels better about everything. She sends the message partly because she wants me to share the moment of freedom.

A negative diagnosis also allows a different relationship to one's child's body and a relaxation of the mothers' anxieties about their babies' bodies. Nonyameko describes how a negative diagnosis allowed the possibility for her daughter's body to become a playful space:

Nonyameko: I, they just told me [my baby is] negative, and I said, 'now my baby can pierce her ears'.

CL: I saw her earrings.

Nonyameko: [laughs] I'm piercing her ears. I did it two days ago; okay now; she didn't get swollen; she didn't have that infection, whatever. So I said, 'okay'.

Nonyameko is permitting an invasion of her daughter's body only because infection is not present. She then observes with delight that her daughter's ears did not become infected. The possibility of infection, it seems, infects everything; any infection may or may not be related to HIV and therefore potentially signals its presence. With the reassurance of its absence, the possibility of a little pus and a little invasion of the body has lost its potential meaning, and Nonyameko's daughter's ears can be pierced. An HIV-negative diagnosis allows a playfulness to emerge in relation to the baby's body and to the mother–infant relationship, quite different to the serious vigilance described before diagnosis.

Relief ameliorates months of uncertainty and vigilance, but what are the implications of having learned to mother a baby under the weight of this uncertainty? Can the matter simply be settled and a new stance towards motherhood adopted? With uncertainty so practised and the stakes so high, it was often difficult for women to simply shift towards certainty. This was particularly the case for the two women whose babies were HIV-positive, who repeatedly, but hopelessly, hoped that a mistake had been made and that their babies would turn out to be negative. A number of women whose babies were diagnosed negative retained the possibility that the doctors had made a mistake and that their babies would in fact turn out to be positive at a later date. Women were told that there was a small possibility that their babies would test falsely negative. For some women, then, there was a small chance that their fears would be confirmed, but even women who had received multiple test results expressed uncertainty about their babies' status.

Boitumelo's story provides one example. Her daughter had been sick and she feared the child may have contracted tuberculosis. The doctors performed thorough examinations, but found no evidence of any disease. Her daughter's HIV test was negative. Her fear that her daughter's sickness may be connected to HIV led her to flatly ignore the negative result:

> *Boitumelo: Ja*, because that time she was sick, you know, so that time she was sick, me, I know I have got that disease, you know? That's why I'm not surprised, you see?

CL: Mm.

Boitumelo: Even the doctors, they can't help me, they can't give me treatment, because they say, 'no, not at this stage'. You see?

CL: Ja.

Boitumelo: That's why they try to check this and this, what's been going on. But they find nothing, you see?

Boitumelo observes her daughter's sickness not through the knowledge of a negative diagnosis, but through the knowledge that 'I have got that disease'. She interprets medical checks as proof that the doctors are searching for HIV, ignoring the fact that they have already made a negative diagnosis. The fact that they 'find nothing' means that they can't find what is there, not that there is nothing to find. The possibility of similarity between mother and daughter is more salient than a medical test. She focuses instead on the need for constant surveillance and on a sense of the powerlessness of the doctors. She does not allow herself to exhale, because the fact of her daughter's ill-health evokes HIV more powerfully than a negative test refutes it, and because believing that her daughter may be positive is easier than acknowledging that her daughter is negative, but fearing that the test could be wrong.

For Palesa, the anxiety of such a possibility never quite went away. Her son, one year old, had tested negative three times (at four months, six months and one year) and was definitely negative. She spoke in our first interview about her relief and about how she used to be 'overprotective' about her son's body, but explained that this had eased as she had become more secure in the fact that he was negative. In the following interview, however, she spoke about her worry that she had found 'enlarged glands' on his body. A doctor had assured her that this was not a sign of HIV infection. Technically, she no longer needed to look for signs, but the visual presence of glands outweighed this knowledge.

CONCLUSION

Examining the emotional resonances of the baby's body for HIV-positive mothers foregrounds the link between the baby and the mother herself. This chapter has focused on the ways in which mothers searched their babies' bodies for clues about whether their babies may have been infected by them and, consequently, for evidence of what kind of mothers they are. The interview material examined in this chapter alternates between proliferations of meaning and loss of words. In the uncertainty of maternal status, knowledge is nebulous – lost and then found, and sometimes lost again. Observing one's baby's body, imagining what might be inside and referring constantly to the possibility of illness intersects both loudly and wordlessly with fantasies of HIV and anxieties about what is inside and what is outside. Within a maternal discourse tinged by the possible associations of HIV-positive motherhood, medical discourse offered both promise and failure; anxieties and fantasies about HIV were both ameliorated and unaffected by the promise of medicine.

Once the wait was over and the baby's status known, the possibility of knowing motherhood became more entrenched. With this, a different kind of potential space opened between baby and mother in which the playfulness and assurance of motherhood could enter. It is quite clear that the long wait before mothers know whether their babies are HIV-positive or -negative intervenes directly in the mother–infant relationship. Technology is rapidly improving to the point that this wait is practically eliminated if one can afford to test earlier. Policy should take seriously that the early mother–infant relationship is important, that the children and future adults of South Africa are severely affected by HIV, and that the statistics clearly indicate that HIV-positive mothers are an important category in their own right. If this is to be acknowledged, then earlier testing of babies becomes an obligation rather than a luxury. This study has suggested that earlier testing may not eliminate the uncertainty characteristic of HIV-positive motherhood, but would certainly have a positive impact on the psychological experiences of both mother and child. A related issue that seems to be absent from public discussion concerns the availability of birth by caesarean section, which further reduces the probability of mother-to-child-transmission, offering women another means of taking control over both motherhood and the virus. This needs to become a real option for all HIV-positive mothers. The fact that knowledge of the baby's status does not eliminate fantasies of infection, however, needs to be acknowledged. Within the context of early HIV-positive motherhood, where so many fantasies can turn into their opposites, it is unsurprising that mothers did not simply abandon fantasies of HIV because of the reality of medical tests. Maternal concern outweighs facts, and loss (including the possibility of loss of identity) has a different relationship to reality in the inner world, particularly when that inner world evokes anxieties and fears echoed in social discourse about the destructiveness of HIV-positive motherhood. For early testing to have a greater impact, some of these associations of HIV-positive motherhood need to be addressed.

The question of the baby's status and the baby's body, then, is partly a question of what the mother has done to the baby, partly of searching the unknown and of confronting the visceral experience of one's baby's body with trepidation, and partly also a question of similarity versus difference between one's baby and oneself. Constructing oneself as a mother involves trying to know what one's baby is and therefore what one is oneself. The baby's body is a site where one's greatest fears (about oneself and one's baby) can be played out, but it also holds potential as a site of salvation. It is a site of multiple conflicts and surrenders in which anxiety hovers, never quite being able to hook onto discourse either to explain, to resist or to reassure. Doctors and medical technology are interspersed through the interview extracts as the primary objects outside the mother and baby; this has been discussed here because precious few other objects were present. The analysis suggests that within the uncertainty of diagnosis, everything can turn into its opposite. This means that everything can be undone, but also that nothing is as it seems. The lack of explanatory frameworks has the quality of foregrounding the raw physical existence of the baby's body. Few elaborate explanations can be voiced; much can be thought, but little concluded. The questions of what to say and what to think are central, but answers are not forthcoming. Within the context of this uncertainty, what does one do in the day-to-day interactional tasks of motherhood? This question is addressed in the next chapter.

6. Mother's Mind

The baby's body does not exist in isolation. In the previous chapter, the meaning of the baby's body was continually processed through the eyes of the mother observing her baby. The baby's body comes into existence through the very physical experience of the mother being pregnant and giving birth. Care of a child, particularly a baby, is intricately involved with holding, handling and feeding. Communication between mother and baby is sensory and physical: motherhood is a bodily experience. In these early stages before language, but also as the child grows, the experience of motherhood is one of imagining oneself into the world of the baby and of holding one's baby in one's fantasies and in one's identity. This is partly what Winnicott means by the phrase 'there is no such thing as a baby'. 'If you set out to describe a baby, you will find that you are describing a *baby and someone*. A baby cannot exist alone, but is essentially part of a relationship' (Winnicott, 1964: 88). Winnicott is suggesting that investigating babyhood can only be done through investigating mother–infant interaction, since it is impossible to separate the two. Similarly, there is no such thing as a mother. If you set out to describe a mother, you must find a mother and baby. Investigating motherhood is incomplete without investigating the mother's experience of the minute communications and occurrences between mother and child, and the ways in which the mother makes sense of her own identity through the relationship she has with her baby. This is at least partly the case because of its importance to mothers; in this study, the mother–infant dyad and maternal care were given more salience than contemplation of meanings of motherhood for the woman herself. Maternal care is as much about the mother's mind as it is about the process of mother minding baby.

This chapter suggests that HIV dominates mothers' interpretations of maternal care, just as in the previous chapter HIV dominated the interpretation of every mark on the baby's body, from diarrhoea to nappy rash to a smile or a pierced ear. It will be suggested in this chapter that fear of infection dominated constructions of motherhood. Many of the normal anxieties of motherhood (Is my baby safe and healthy? Am I a good mother? Will my baby love me? Will I damage my baby?) were channelled almost exclusively into HIV-related anxiety. Each question that mothers normally ask was reframed in relation to infection. The continual searching of the mother's mind described in this chapter has a particular quality of obsessiveness. Mother–infant interaction invokes anxieties about what kind of mother one is, as well as what kind of baby one has: two people are involved. The HIV-positive mother is left with a certain breathlessness and lack of words, because discourse cannot contain the anxiety of infection. Questions regarding one's baby are different to questions regarding oneself. The HIV-positive person looks at herself and asks, 'What does my body mean? Why is my body like this? What can I do? Who am I?'. Questions about the baby are more elusive and floating: 'Is my baby safe? What have I done? Where is s/he? Where am I?.' Being an HIV-positive mother to a baby is spatial and interrelational; HIV is interstitial, invisibly present in between mother and baby.

In this sense, HIV asserts itself into the space between mother and baby, as well as into the subjectivity of the HIV-positive mother. The physicality of the early mother–infant relationship was often defined and directed by fear and uncertainty regarding infection in relation to the literal and metaphoric closeness of mother–infant interaction. This chapter explores common experiences and anxieties of motherhood that have become magnified and colonised by HIV. Further, this is not necessarily explicit and articulated, but often unspoken, sometimes unspeakable, and 'it' exists in day-to-day care – in holding, observing, playing, feeding – as much as in reflections on the meanings of HIV for the mother–infant dyad.

MATERNAL ATTENTIVENESS

Maternal vigilance of the baby's body was similarly described in relation to day-to-day care of the baby. Women often described themselves as 'overprotective' and felt that they needed to execute the daily tasks of motherhood with great attentiveness. Kuli would not let anyone bath her baby; Lesedi refused to let anyone else hold her baby; Amara carefully observed her baby even while the baby slept and did not want to leave her alone for a moment. Two stories will be explored here that illustrate the punctuation of mother–infant interaction by HIV. Lukanyo's story is about feeding her child; Dikeledi's is about keeping her child safe from germs. They provide extreme examples of the attentiveness with which women described caring for their babies, chosen because in their extremity they expose the power of the anxieties experienced by HIV-positive motherhood.

Lukanyo
We begin with Lukanyo, who carefully fed her child and saw his fat body as a sign that he was HIV-negative, referring frequently to his weight as a sign of his health. This also became an important barometer of the mother–infant relationship. When I ask her how things have been going between her and her baby in our third interview, for example, she selects his weight out of all the possible answers she could have given in order to express her pleasure:

No he's growing very, very well .... He was very big, *ja*, at one month. He was very big .... Before he finished one month he was already weighing 6 [kg]. So he was very big .... He's got a lot of good weight, and he looks well; he doesn't look sick.

This is Lukanyo's immediate response to a question about their relationship. Feeding her baby was a means by which she could keep him healthy, ward off infection and look at him in order to find a baby who looks healthy: 'he doesn't look sick.' Being good at feeding her baby translated into being a good mother through protecting her baby from HIV.

Lukanyo shared her concern and pride with many women interviewed. She stood out, however, because her baby was seriously overweight. At two months his weight was equivalent to a seven month old. Her doctors had warned her that she should 'stop feeding so much'. Despite this warning, Lukanyo frequently stated proudly that his weight was a sign of his health and her good motherhood. Doctors' concerns were dismissed, perhaps because these concerns were not about HIV: 'They say if he's four months, I won't be able to carry him [laughs]. Ah, he's fine now, he's fine. He's growing fast [talks to the baby]. He can hold things now. He's growing fast.'

Lukanyo laughs at medical concern; the fact that her baby is much bigger than expected for his age is something that she can take credit for. When her laughter is finished, medical concern is immediately discredited by her own knowledge – and pride – of her baby: 'he's fine ... he's growing'. His weight is equated with his motor development ('he can hold things now') and therefore with normality.

In order to appreciate the importance to Lukanyo of keeping her baby fat and healthy, it is necessary to contextualise her attentiveness in her story of infection and motherhood. Lukanyo believes that she was infected when she was 18 years old. She had met her first boyfriend and was still a virgin, but her mother disapproved and forced her to leave home. She went to live with her boyfriend, because she had nowhere else to go. Feeling indebted to him, she felt she could not refuse him sex. He initially used a condom, but then refused. She left him after a few weeks. She describes becoming sick and losing weight very quickly and was diagnosed HIV-positive the following year. After her diagnosis, she met her second boyfriend and decided that she wanted to have a child before she died. Being unemployed, she could not afford artificial insemination, so made herself gain weight and then used a syringe to get pregnant without putting her boyfriend at risk of HIV infection.

Lukanyo wanted me to tell this story so that people would know that her mother was to blame for her infection, and also that it is possible to choose to become pregnant without the help of the state or medicine and without putting one's partner's life at risk. Her decision to fall pregnant was described as a defiance of social convention, against the medical establishment who would not help her and against the infection itself. The decision symbolised a refusal to allow infection to change her life course; a refusal to allow it to infect her creativity. She was determined to be a good mother to her baby and to show that, despite being rejected by family and community, 'you can have some other things that you want'.

Lukanyo's concern about her baby's weight resonates with at least two aspects of her story. Firstly, her narrative is one of being out of control, of having tragedy befall her through the uncaring actions of others and then of bravely fighting back. This is operationalised on her body through her description of sudden weight loss, and then later a stubborn rejection of her circumstances and her infection by forcing herself to gain weight in order to maximise her chances of falling pregnant. This weight gain symbolises a transition from when 'I was just useless' to a life-saving point at which 'my life is going to change'; it represents her direct challenge to the virus and the people who betrayed her. In this sense, her baby's weight gain is not only a symbol of what she wants for her baby; it is also a point of identification and physical proof that 'I am a fighter, because I've made it through'. It is as much about her own identity as it is about her baby's: her ability to gain weight in order to get pregnant was echoed in her ability to make her baby gain weight and be healthy.

Secondly, Lukanyo knew of her HIV status before falling pregnant; she knew there was a possibility of infecting her baby, but decided that this was a risk worth taking. The decision to have a child knowing one is positive was strongly condemned by all the women in the study,[1] and evokes questions about maternal blameworthiness. In our first interview, Lukanyo's proud and defiant tone presided until I asked her what she thought about her baby's possible HIV status. At this point, tears sprang to her eyes and her voice softened. Imagining her baby as positive,

> I will take it that that means that is the way God wanted my life to be …. But I have tried to change my life. That was the only thing that I was trying to do. Bringing somebody in this world, in this situation, I was trying to make myself happy and I know that I was hurting that person, because of nobody would like to be born in this situation, you see. That was the decision that I took by myself. So I won't be angry that much, I will just take it that that is the way my life was going to be. That means, I was gonna be miserable for the rest of my life.

Lukanyo is prepared to take the chance in the hope of changing her life. It is possible that, within the mother–infant relationship, her fervent feeding of her baby and admiration of her baby's 'good weight' represents an overcompensation for the guilt that she may have infected her baby. Her ability as a mother to facilitate his growth outweighed medical opinion and served as a defence against HIV infection and her fears that her baby would die. Feeding her baby helped to keep him healthy, but also became a symbolic shield against the infection of his body and against her fears about his status.

Dikeledi

Dikeledi's concern is not with her baby's weight, but with what goes in and out of his body. She ruefully describes herself as an 'overprotective' mother

---

1   Including Lukanyo herself, as the next chapter will demonstrate.

and deprecatingly describes her hypervigilance regarding her son when he was smaller. Other children spent much time around her son, but they were so aware of her overprotectiveness that they knew they were not allowed to touch him or kiss him, in case they gave him any 'germs'. When they needed to cough, they were instructed to do so far away from him. She remembers them making fun of her, standing far away and coughing loudly while they laughingly told her that they were not near her baby. Other mothers similarly went to extreme measures to keep their babies safe from 'dirt' or 'germs'. Dikeledi's description vividly portrays how HIV intervenes in the holding of the baby – in the kiss or the cuddle. This was also the case with her own holding of her baby:

> He knows that whenever he gets sick, I just spoil him; I just hold him; I don't do anything. I just, you know, whenever he sleeps … I wouldn't sleep when he used to sleep, uh-uh, I would just hold him. Whenever he cries, whenever he coughs, I would just jump.

Dikeledi describes a watchfulness common to many mothers, but her vigilance is not just for her baby's comfort. Her care of her baby's sickness or cry or cough is a protection against HIV. If she lets her guard down for a moment, infection might take over.

Dikeledi identifies this overprotection as one of the ways in which she is a 'bad mother'. Her description of watchfulness despite concern about being overprotective resonates with other stories. Her story stands out, not only for her ability to teach other children to stay away from her baby, but also in the fact that this overprotectiveness did not go away after her son was diagnosed HIV-negative. Her 11-month-old son had been diagnosed negative for over seven months, but 'I'm still quite protective. I'm more protective than anything'. Her son is crawling and learning to walk, and, typically, wants to put everything into his mouth. Dikeledi describes, however, that she has taught him so well that he never actually puts anything into his mouth. When he picks something up and brings it towards his mouth, he looks at her and puts it down again. She says that when she gives him a cheese curl, he will wait for her to put it into his mouth before he knows he can eat it. 'You know he, he knows, "I want to take to the mouth, but I can't take it to the mouth". *Ja.* That's what I do.' Although her son is HIV-negative, Dikeledi continues to monitor what goes into his body. Her fear of infection is such that he has learned not to put anything in his mouth without her permission – quite an achievement for an 11-month-old baby. In the daily practice of motherhood, her fear outweighs the relief that her baby is negative.

Lukanyo and Dikeledi illustrate broader processes of watchfulness in the daily tasks of motherhood and each suggests something of the anxieties associated with caring for a potentially HIV-positive baby. Lukanyo's desire to keep her baby fat illustrates the desire to be a good mother in order to protect her baby's health, as well as the guilt of possibly being the bad infecting mother. Dikeledi's 'overprotectiveness' of her baby illustrates the danger of a potentially infectious world, which, for her, does not go away even after her baby is pronounced safe.

THE INTERRUPTION OF THE MOTHER–INFANT RELATIONSHIP BY HIV

Maternal attentiveness, then, is constructed in the service of protecting a child against the ever present possibility of infection as well as in the service of protecting one's own subjectivity and the threats of guilt and death that assail it. Surveillance of infection was particularly described in relation to maternal care of the baby's body, as the examples above illustrate, but also erupted at unexpected moments.

Two examples from Ayanda's interviews will illustrate how easily holding one's child in one's mind can summon fantasies of infection. In the first example, Ayanda has spent an intimate moment talking to her baby, then looks up at me and says:

∽

He's such a nice child. He's so nice; he doesn't cry; he's always happy. Even when he got that flu, I went to the doctor and the doctor said, 'but this child doesn't look sick'. I said, 'haai, this child is sick'.

In contemplating how 'nice' her baby is, the possibility of sickness immediately arises. The 'nice' child is counterposed against the 'sick' child. The speed at which she moves from existing together with and admiring her child to sickness seems to suggest that fears about her baby's health are close to the surface. Similarly, in the second example, Ayanda is proudly explaining to me why she chose her baby's name, which means 'blessing', and in this moment of pride thinks about his new achievements:

Ayanda: He's trying to, to crawl. He's, you know, he can't stay on one position when he's sleeping, especially with the tummy. He gets there [laughs]. I'm glad some of the babies, most of them here have tested, eh, negative. Mm. [talks to and plays with the baby for a while]. You know, there's something wrong here, Carol. It makes like a lump there.

CL: Is that his inoculation?

Ayanda: Yes. Oh, you still, you know, with the babies, né, you look, maybe it's one of the AIDS symptoms, and you're always looking so carefully; you want to find the wrong thing and fortunately you can't find anything.

Her baby's new achievement brings joyful laughter at his developmental progression ('he gets there') and then immediately brings his status into question, in the form of the hope that he, like other babies, may end up being HIV-negative. After a moment of interaction, her play with her baby turns into the now familiar scanning of his body for signs of infection. Perhaps he is HIV-positive? What does this lump mean (a lump common when children are inoculated)? HIV sneaks up and takes over the playful space between mother and child.

A typical mother–infant interaction turned into a search for HIV for Boitumelo as well. During one of our interviews, her baby started crying and she realised that she had forgotten her bottle at home. Her baby became increasingly distressed and Boitumelo could not calm her. She tried to feed her, but she would not take the food. Boitumelo became visibly distressed as her baby continued crying, saying that this was the first time that she had ever left her bottle at home. When her baby eventually settled, she spoke about her guilt that she had forgotten her baby's bottle when her baby could so easily become sick.

> *Boitumelo:* So I think, 'shame', you know, 'she's crying'; I forgot the bottle, you see?
> *CL: Ja.*
> *Boitumelo: Ja,* it's not good …. The doctors can think I don't feed this baby.

Boitumelo's guilt at having forgotten her baby's bottle makes her worry about how the doctors (and perhaps I) will perceive her as a mother. Her fear is that she will be labelled neglectful, and perhaps her guilt about her oversight makes her feel like this. Once the baby settles, though, she can immediately go back to describing her conversations with the doctor in which her baby was proclaimed healthy: 'but if you will hear the doctor, you see now she's okay. Now she's okay.' The unsettled baby opens the door for infection; as the baby settles, the door can be closed.

Ayanda and Boitumelo are caught unawares by infection. Each of them is simply spending time caring for her baby, doing the things that normal mothers do – admiring motor development, worrying when the baby cries, hoping everything will be well. Within moments, something reminds them about HIV and this comes to the foreground, subsuming other hopes and fears. Everything always comes back to HIV.

The loss of breastfeeding

It is possible that Boitumelo's guilt at having forgotten her baby's bottle is linked to one of the most visible symbols of HIV in mother–infant interaction: the fact that she was not breastfeeding, because of her fear that her baby may 'drink the disease'. Boitumelo was very matter-of-fact about the absolute imperative not to breastfeed. Whether or not her lack of breastfeeding fuelled her distress at having forgotten her baby's bottle remains conjecture. She was not interested in discussing this; her decision not to breastfeed was simply a requirement. Breastfeeding was frequently discussed and experienced as a powerful reminder of the presence of HIV within the mother–infant dyad, particularly because so many women were criticised by others for being bad mothers (and bad cultural members) because they did not breastfeed. Despite this, all the women were adamant about their decision not to breastfeed, often in a similarly matter-of-fact and curt manner to Boitumelo. When contemplating what her decision means for her, Joyce says, 'I don't feel nothing, because I know that, *eish*, it's the best thing I can do [pause]. Because it is not going to help if I just breastfeed'. She allows no possibility for feeling regret at her decision, because it is too important to remain steadfast. So too with Petunia:

Ah, mm, I don't have a problem [with breastfeeding], *ja*, I don't have a problem because I said, if that time when I said I'm going to take a blood, if that time I had said I don't want, now I'm having her, if that time I had said I don't want, now my baby, what is going to happen with my baby? So I feel happy, I feel happy, I feel happy. Serious.

In between 'I don't have a problem' and 'I feel happy' lies a possible explanation as to why it is so important to give an adamant response. Petunia's explanation is shrouded in vagueness and generality, but she has decided what she *wants* and therefore has the responsibility of protecting her baby from further possibilities of infection. Her eloquence fails at the point of trying to put the threat into words; her repetition of 'I feel happy' is about her refusal to breastfeed and therefore her choice to counteract this threat. Lukanyo is as adamant, but refers more directly to the threat:

> *Lukanyo:* No I'm not going to breastfeed. No I am not.
> *CL:* Why not, for you?
> *Lukanyo:* No, ... it's fine not to breastfeed, because of, like, I know that I have this disease, and have to try to protect; they say you must protect the one you love. So if I breastfeed, that means I wanted to kill that child. So I don't wanted to kill this, my child, I just want to be happy; I just wanted to see my child being healthy like other kids. So I'm not going to breastfeed. Well, it's not nice not to breastfeed, especially us blacks; you know. If you don't breastfeed, there is, that is another thing.

Lukanyo's decision against breastfeeding is a matter of life and death, which overrides both her sacrifice and cultural criticism. It becomes a symbol of love and protection, proof that she is a good mother, and a powerful antidote to the thought of her child's death. It also offers a defence against maternal guilt. Lukanyo, like Zodwa, does not want to be responsible for her own child's death. Zodwa's decision not to breastfeed protects her from compounding guilt:

> I don't want to blame myself, when he's positive, he must be positive, as, as from giving birth, not like here, feeding. Like not saying, 'oh, it was my fault again'. No. I don't want to feel guilty; I don't want to blame myself again.

Zodwa's comments indicate the power of guilt in the mother–infant relationship. Her 'again' makes it clear that she is not just concerned about the possibility of infecting her baby. She is concerned about a repetition of failure as a mother, a repetition of being infectious and blameworthy. Refusal to breastfeed offers some power, but it is not an uncomplicated symbol of love, protection and good motherhood.

The decision not to breastfeed represents a choice to save one's baby, but because mother's milk is highly valued, it also has a reverse meaning: that women are depriving their children of something crucial. Dikeledi's longing to be able to breastfeed prompts her to ask others what it feels like:

[B]ecause it's nice and it's like you are bonding with the baby, so, like, I feel that, you know, I never got a chance to breastfeed my baby, give him proper nutritions and everything, so I bond with him while he's being fed. *Ja*, that's the thing. 'Cos, like, I had to use a bottle feed.

There is a dual loss implicit in her description: firstly, a loss of being able to do her best for her baby and the awful feeling that bonding and nutrition are compromised, and, secondly, a loss of feeling the joy of this aspect of mother–infant interaction.

Talk about breastfeeding raised fears about the adequacy of the attachment between mother and child. This was often described with an attentiveness and devotion similar to descriptions of other aspects of the baby's care. Thandiwe gives a typical description of how she tries very hard to mimic the breastfeeding situation and to create an intimate space between mother and baby:

You just take your baby and put her here [next to her bosom] and you just looking her over on her eyes and she just looks you on your eyes. As you are breastfeeding, she's here, just looking here, you see. The thing that, it's just a baby, even if you breastfeed or not, you just have to give the baby that love, *ja*.

Thandiwe has thought about how to compensate for her lack of breastfeeding and has carefully utilised this in her interaction with her baby. This place of calm offers some kind of completion and a visual, physical sense of being a mother to a baby. Thandiwe does not explicitly refer here to the reasons for its importance, but, as with the decision not to breastfeed, the creation of a space in which to bond is important precisely because of the infection lurking on its edges. Tumi refers more directly to this fear:

> I sometimes wish to give her my breast, you know. But I become so scared, yo, because what if I give my baby anything, she become so infected, you know, so I gave her the bottle. You know, when you breastfeed a child, there is that communication. It happens just like, bottle, she has to touch my face, you know, kick with her feet, and I would talk to her and look; she'll look at me very closely, you know. And that's part of the, maybe it's our bond, it's how we respond to each other.

Tumi also longs to breastfeed and worries about the impact of not breastfeeding on communication between mother and child, but her fear of infection is greater. She counterpoints this fear and longing, as well as the risk to communication, against the charm of the mother–infant feeding situation. Here, mother and baby become involved in a communication that, in its involvement and exclusivity, keeps infection firmly on the edges and creates something unique: 'our bond.'

While most women split off the bad parts of their decision not to breastfeed as firmly as possible, it is clear that the consequences for mothers of breastfeeding are not as straightforward as just being 'happy'. Zinzi, who also tries to create an exclusive space between herself and her baby, gives the matter-of-fact answer to the question of breastfeeding:

> I am not breastfeeding at all. I am giving a bottle. Because I thought maybe it was the same with breastfeeding and you've got this disease, you see; I think that when you give him the bottle, it is the best way. Mm.

She cannot, however, quite eject the awfulness of her loss of breastfeeding. I ask her what this has meant for her:

Zinzi: Hey, it is bad. When I saw, when I go to the clinic, I saw
someone who is breastfeeding her baby, hey, I am feeling so bad
that, that maybe I am not the mother that want to give the best
for the baby, for, for, for her baby. I really feel bad.

CL: How do you think you have managed bonding with your baby?

Zinzi: Oh. Hey [sighs and laughs]. It was tough for me, because I
think that sometimes I don't have a baby at all, you see. I feel, I
feel that knock because I don't breastfeed my baby. I feel distant
between me and him. Even if when I am giving him the bottle, I
feel distance, I start to think, it's this distance between us. But then
for the best, [sighs] I have to give him the bottle.

It is difficult for Zinzi to feel like a mother, particularly when she compares
herself to breastfeeding mothers. This feels like both an internal gap and
an external gap between herself and her baby. When contemplating her
comments in light of the quotations above, the existence of HIV in the
space between mother and baby becomes more concretely spatial; one can
almost imagine it as a physical object occupying space, always on the edges,
sometimes elbowing its way through to centre stage. Lungile talks about
the struggle in space between herself and her baby: her baby seeks out her
breast and she has to refuse, although it is 'hard to resist'. She resists because
HIV is in between her breast and her baby's mouth; she has no choice.

Lungile's guilt at withholding, however, at one point makes a mockery
of her resolve. She has decided not to breastfeed 'because of my sickness',
but in a moment of worry, this logic comes undone. She contemplates
the fact that her child has been sick and immediately feels guilty: 'Even
that time he was sick, I thought, "if I was breastfeeding him, he wouldn't
be sick".' The logic of protecting him from sickness by not breastfeeding
turns into its opposite – that her decision has jeopardised his health, not
protected it. She is left in an impossible situation.

The steadfastness with which women refused to breastfeed, as with
the attentiveness with which they carried out the tasks of motherhood, is

clearly not without conflict and contradiction. The strength of resolve to be a caring and vigilant mother who attends superbly to her baby's needs illustrated above seems to act as a barrier against infection, as well as against maternal guilt and the spectre of death. The analysis suggests, however, that infection recursively undermines resolve. Contradiction, uncertainty and doubt erode this resolve, while the persistence of infection, which serves to strengthen it, is such that determination is never strong enough. The mother–infant relationship is always under threat and HIV silently exists in between the (not) nursing mother and her baby. HIV occupies this minimal space in this '(not)' and in the blood ties between mother and baby, where the possibility of infection is itself infectious. In the desperate attempt to contain it in the mother–baby relationship, through the mother's containment of the baby's body and the mother's mind, infection symbolically proliferates and spreads, taking fear and guilt along with it.

CONCLUSION

The concentration and care with which women engaged with early motherhood suggest that women were particularly motivated to make the most out of early mother–infant attachment. Since this period is largely considered to be crucial for later mental health, it offers the potential for mother and baby to build a solid relational foundation. This seems particularly important, given that children of HIV-positive mothers are likely to lose their mothers at some point and are also increasingly likely to survive themselves, as prevention of mother-to-child-transmission becomes more readily available. The honesty and sophistication with which women engaged in research interviews in this study further suggest that systems of support for the mother–infant dyad would be of benefit to the mother as well as the baby. If such support systems were in place, and were able to tolerate the pain and uncertainty of this period of motherhood, as well as able to tolerate understandings of HIV-positive maternity as important for both baby and mother, it appears likely that mothers would be able to use the support to help them to tolerate their own pain and uncertainty and their own desires to be good mothers.

In the foregoing analysis, steadfastness, fear and guilt have been firmly located in the mother's mind, and few other objects in the social world have been examined. This reflects the extent to which such objects were absent in discussion of the mother–infant relationship, although present elsewhere. The exclusivity of the relationship, perhaps, left little room in the mothers' minds for anything else. This exclusivity is evident in the ways in which the mothers spoke about their babies, but also in the infrequency with which other people were spoken about. It was clear that other caregivers were present in everyday life. These were sometimes dual mothers and sometimes competitors, but their day-to-day functions were relatively absent from the discussion, with caregiving responsibility belonging exclusively to the mother. Fathers had little contact with the mother–infant dyad; those who were present were generally constructed as fathers only in name. The women seldom engaged in discussion about the impact of fatherhood on their partners, and almost never about the practice of fatherhood. When questions about fathers were asked, the prototypical response was, 'he's fine'. The women wanted their babies to be with them and constructed themselves solitarily as caregivers.

With steadfastness, fear and guilt located in the mother's mind, infection was firmly located in the baby. When the women positioned themselves as mothers concerned about infection of their baby, their own position of infected person was seldom visited. Within the individuality of the mother–infant relationship, something feels natural about the exclusivity of the mother's emotions and concerns for her baby's infection. In discussing mother and baby, the fact that a social analysis is difficult to find seems to make sense. It is almost as if there is no need. However, the mother's guilt, for example, is not just a personal feeling. It is an affect very much connected to broader social constructions of motherhood. The extent to which guilt played a role in the analysis reflects the incorporation of social expectations into subjectivity. Similarly, the selflessness of focus on the baby's infection and the overwhelming desire to be a good mother is also connected to expectations regarding the perfection of motherhood. When Neo worries that 'I am not the mother who want to give the best for the baby', she is drawing directly on such constructions. Focus on the innocent baby's body and the mother's efficacy seems only fair, at least from within shared constructions of motherhood in which a mother is a mother of a baby. However, when seeking out the mother's body in the following chapter, the neutrality of the focus on the baby loses some of its transparency, and one realises the extent to which discourses of motherhood make their mark.

7. Mother's Body

∞

Motherhood is dominantly a secondary identity in which the baby is more important than the mother. It seems that adding HIV to the mix explodes this expectation of facelessness. Although interview material was predominantly concerned with motherhood from the perspective of the baby, there were notable instances where women occupied motherhood *from their own perspectives*. This chapter examines some such moments, focusing particularly on the maternal body. This body, which belongs only to the mother and which expresses the feelings and identities of maternity, signifies one place where motherhood lives in its own right. The previous chapters suggested that the baby's body – its meaning, status and the care it receives in mother–infant interaction – is central to HIV-positive motherhood. In its urgency, it drowns out the mother's body. Examining the ways in which the mother's body entered (or did not enter) into interviews – providing an analysis of the margins that support the centre, or of the bodily container that holds motherhood as well as babyhood – makes it easier to recognise the power and pervasiveness of dominant discourses about motherhood, which posit the all-importance of the baby and, implicitly, the absence of the mother. Analysing the few and very specific instances where the mother's body did emerge in interviews also foregrounds the ways in which these dominant discourses police the boundaries of subjectivity. The mother's body does not only foreground dominant discourses, however; its existence, sidelined as it is, also challenges them. The mother's body cannot be made sufficiently docile, and so breaks through and threatens (at the boundaries of subjectivity) the dominance of discourses that the mother's body and the mother's identity are fundamentally less important than the baby.

This chapter suggests that, while the maternal body is largely absent from interview material, it nonetheless inserts itself – and maternal identity – in important moments. These moments are entangled with HIV-positive identities: the mother's body is most visible as an infecting body; it is most powerfully evoked through the stories of other HIV-positive mothers; it is constructed and reconstructed through the baby's HIV status. Such moments also participate in the splits found in dominant conceptions of HIV-positive motherhood. The maternal body is thereby unsettled in the perpetual question regarding whether it is a good body or a bad body. As Melanie Klein's paranoid-schizoid baby is obsessed alternately and separately with the good and bad breast, so the mother's body, from her own perspective, shifts between good and bad, sometimes settling in the differently uncomfortable position that it is both. Nevertheless, these almost-silenced moments where the maternal body was visible and present highlight the spaces through which maternal identity challenges the all-importance of the baby and the invisibility of the mother herself to suggest the gaps between fantasies of HIV-positive motherhood and embodied experience.

THE LARGELY ABSENT MOTHER'S BODY

Where is the mother's body? The short answer is given by Nombeko. She is describing how her stiff body or the feeling that her 'eyesight is getting shorter' leads her immediately to her HIV-positive body and the fear of HIV: 'ooh, I think it's working; it's doing it's job now.' In a moment of reflection on her body as a mother's body, she then speaks as follows:

> *Nombeko:* You know, I don't take it that much as a mother's body. I just take the way, [pause] *ja.*
> *CL:* It's kind of more about the HIV in your body?
> *Nombeko:* Yes. Yes.

Nombeko cannot identify her maternal body with herself, because HIV – which in the moment of articulation cannot be put into words (as the pause indicates) – has taken over. When bodies were spoken about in interviews, this was overwhelmingly in relation either to the baby's body or to the woman's body as an HIV-positive person – ungendered, desexualised and certainly not the body of a mother. When motherhood was under discussion, the primary body was the baby's; when the woman herself was the subject, the primary body was HIV-positive. All the interviews were characterised by this split, and the women often moved from one conversation to the next – from being an HIV-positive person to a baby's mother – as if from one continent to another.

Yet motherhood is a very bodily enterprise. As one moves into the identity of motherhood, a number of bodily changes occur. Pregnancy transforms one's body; birth is profoundly physical; caring for a baby is a bodily experience, e.g. of touching and smelling, of one's bodily recovery after labour, of getting too little sleep, hormonal changes, carrying a baby, and one's reduced opportunity to care for one's body (Pines, 1993). The maternal body is something that mothers frequently want to discuss and that holds complex meanings for their sense of identity (Raphael-Leff, 1991). There was almost no talk in interviews about these more directly physical experiences. A minority of women mentioned, for example, the experience of their bodies becoming larger in the last stages of pregnancy or their breasts being sore from not being able to breastfeed. These comments, however, were fleeting, mostly before or after interviews, almost as if discussing the weather, and quickly dismissed.

On a more psychological level, women often experience the bodily changes of motherhood as a transformation or attack on their identity and on their autonomy as separate beings (Parker, 1995). The practice of motherhood can mean having to make one's body secondary, having it 'owned' by one's baby. Pregnancy itself reshapes one's body, and it is very common for women to experience pregnancy as an invasion of their bodies, entertaining, for example, fantasies of parasitic take-over or that a foreign object is depleting their bodies (Raphael-Leff, 1993; Pines, 1997). This can often be difficult for women to admit to, and even more difficult to accept, given the power of idealisations of motherhood (Parker, 1995), but frequently surfaces. Despite the frankness of the women in this study about their fears and fantasies regarding their own and their babies' bodies, those connected to the mothers' bodies were notably absent from interviews. In terms of explicit reference, it was almost as if the body had no category related to 'mother'.

Does this mean that the mother's body does not exist in this particular context of HIV-positive motherhood? Has that aspect of motherhood belonging most clearly only to the mother been written out of experience? I would like to suggest that the object of the mother's body is not simply absent from discourse, but rather that it cannot be acknowledged (at least directly) as of importance. An extract from an interview with Bongiwe, in which she does not directly talk about her body as a mother's, helps to illustrate and introduce the spectral presence of the mother's body and some possibilities regarding the threat it poses and the need for it to be hidden. I will present the entire interchange and then suggest that the threat of her body can be read into her topic changes and their relationship to different kinds of anxieties, as well as to two different kinds of babies.

In our second interview, Bongiwe talks about recent test results that confirm her baby is HIV-positive. At one point, she speaks with frustration about having taken Nevirapine and having abstained from breastfeeding, but that these preventative measures do not seem to have worked. At this point, she is the infecting mother and her baby the infected baby. I say to her, 'It's hard, hey?'. She responds: 'And to all of my kids; they are saying that this one, she's very pretty than the others, but she's the one who gave me sickness than the others.'

Her baby has shifted from infected to infecting baby. She then says that she chose her baby's name because it means 'answer'.

> *Bongiwe:* Because I was praying for her, I was praying because I was very sick, but it was not from her. From the HIV. The child was inside, so I was not feeling well, so I was just praying, 'let this kid, let this, when it comes to the world, let it be alive'. So I was praying, I was praying and then after giving birth, then the baby was alive, then I said, 'no, let it be the answer'.
>
> *CL:* And that's [her name]?
>
> *Bongiwe:* Yes, it's [her name] .... This means 'answer', even if we are praying and ask for something and it came exactly the way you asked. So her father wanted her name to be Julia, so I don't know what Julia means. Do you?
>
> *CL:* I don't know what Julia means.
>
> *Bongiwe:* And it's hard, because it is his first baby. So I don't know whether the others are going to be like, but I don't want to have a baby anymore. But I pray that maybe if he is having a baby, let it be mine again. If he keeps on giving, he's going to spread AIDS.

The interchange begins with Bongiwe contemplating the most frightening link between her body and her baby's – that the mother's body transmitted the virus to her baby. Her own body is not directly invoked, but its implied presence is as both an HIV-positive body and a mother's body. In the pain of the possibility of infection, Bongiwe changes the subject to a consideration of how her other children evaluate this baby as different, because the baby is pretty (Bongiwe's body has produced something beautiful), but 'she's the one who gave me sickness'. As she moves to the issue of her baby's name (her baby's identity), this remarkable reversal that the baby infected the mother remains unelaborated. Bongiwe attributes this logic to her other two children, not to herself. Whether or not her children said this (which is unlikely: she has repeatedly stressed that she is too fearful to tell anyone, including her children, about her status), the reversal comes to her mind and is then undone at this particular point in the interview. Its slipperiness suggests her fantasy that the baby gave her HIV, not the other way around. In this formulation (and Bongiwe was not the only woman to formulate this), the moment of conception is the moment of HIV – baby and virus are simultaneous, and it is the baby, not the mother, who is destructive. Bongiwe's interchange begins with her fear of having infected her baby, which is then transformed into, perhaps projected onto, her baby as infectious. The moment when the woman's body becomes a mother's body is the moment that it also becomes an HIV-positive body.

This foregrounds an obvious fact about any mother's body: her existence as mother is proof that she has had sex, a fact that is subject to widespread cultural denial. The existence of HIV provides further proof of sexuality, but with very different social connotations. The mother's body becomes double proof of sex, through the existence of the baby as well as of the virus. In this brief moment in Bongiwe's interview ('she's the one who gave me sickness'), her body is not directly present. It has been made to disappear along with its power to infect. It is suggested that the seeming absence of the mother's body from the interviews represents, at least in part, a distancing from the sexuality and infection that this body so dangerously evokes.

As Bongiwe shifts from 'she's the one who gave me sickness' to 'answer', she undoes the fantasy of the infecting baby and perhaps the anxiety of her sexual and infecting maternal body by foregrounding her baby's identity, as well as herself in choosing this visionary and optimistic name. Put differently, she moves from a position in which she is HIV-positive *because* of motherhood to a position of motherhood in which her creativity and identity coexist with the identity of her baby, and which implies the defeat of HIV (and the reparation of her own destructiveness), or the *answer* to HIV, through her creativity (her creation of both the name and her baby).

She then moves to her own body ('I was very sick'). In so doing, she evokes the mother's body with the 'child inside', but simultaneously denies its existence: 'it was not from her. From the HIV.' She is saying that her child did *not* make her sick, and in order to do that, her body is constructed as HIV-positive and *not* a mother's body. Her shift away from the position of motherhood towards HIV allows her to undo the fantasy that her baby has infected her. The anxiety that follows this shift has to do with the fear that her baby may be dead: 'let it be alive.' The mother's body is dismissed in relation to the fear that the mother's body is infecting.

The relief that 'the baby was alive' allows her to be a mother again, because her prayers saved her baby: 'it came out exactly the way you asked.' But this leads her to the third and hidden player in her baby's infection, her husband. Bongiwe believes that she was infected by her husband; this, then, is the reason she passed infection on to her baby. Significantly, the mother's body was kept entirely separate from the gendered body throughout the interviews; similarly, discussions of motherhood were not connected with the presence of the father. This is one of the few instances where the partner's role as father was spontaneously acknowledged. Her husband is immediately reconstructed, however, from father ('it is his first baby') through her fear of her body making her a mother again ('I don't want to have a baby anymore') to impregnating man. She does not want to be a mother again, but she prays that if he has another baby, he keeps infection in the family. This highlights two aspects of the mother's body common across interviews that perhaps contribute to its seeming absence. Firstly, the mother's body is kept isolated from the bodies of other adults, but particularly from her partner (whether he is absent or present), and this suggests not only anxiety attached to the mother's body, but also to the means by which it was itself infected. Secondly, the maternal body is capable of making another baby. Bongiwe does not directly say why she does not want another baby (this unelaborated adamance was repeated by almost all the women interviewed), but the implication of the threat of infection and of 'spread' is clear. To acknowledge the mother's body means to acknowledge its ability both to procreate and to destroy and be destroyed.

This very short interchange illustrates the ways in which the mother's body only occupied the margins of discussion, but was far from absent or irrelevant in interviews. The seeming absence indicates not a lack, but an excess of meaning. In essence, then, the mother's body was absent because this body excludes HIV and it excludes the baby. At the same time, it is a powerful reminder of infection, of powerlessness to protect self and baby, of sexuality and of potential destruction. It is suggested that being an HIV-positive mother within a very powerful discursive field prompts the imperative to construct one's body as desexualised. Linked to this, the mother's body evokes the ability to procreate, which again evokes the threat of infection and death. Attention now turns to analysis of places in interviews in which the mother's body was directly visible.

THE MOTHER'S BODY POWERFULLY EVOKED AS AN INFECTING BODY

A possible reason for the absence of the mother's body is that it is spun around the nucleus of guilt regarding possible infection of the baby by the mother. This directly evokes the HIV-positive body as a mother's body: in this way, the mother's body cannot be ignored. Dominant constructions in interviews were that the body of the HIV-positive person is infected; the body of the HIV-positive mother is infecting. It is therefore significant that there was considerable silence about the bodily mechanisms of the ways in which mothers infect babies – that the infecting mother was seldom directly imagined.

The three instances connected with bodily functions and motherhood represent exceptions in interview material, but their visual power is striking. Firstly, and most commonly, there was a fear of one's own death during delivery. Before Bongiwe gave birth, for example, she was scared she would not survive the birth of her baby. Thandiwe, interviewed on the day she was due to give birth, was terrified that she would die that day. This fear suggests the destruction of the mother's body by the act of becoming a mother. It is a fear shared by many mothers, HIV-positive or not (Pines, 1993); in this case, it was inflected by HIV in two possible ways: firstly, when this common fear did surface in interviews, it was translated exclusively through the lens of HIV. This was not the common fear of not surviving the birth process, but the fear of not surviving *because* of the existence of HIV in the body. Secondly, although more common than the instances to follow, it was still very seldom voiced and, when so, dismissed with speed. Thandiwe perhaps expressed this fear most powerfully because of the proximity of the birth process, but she did so only after the interview had finished, once it was 'off record'. The paucity of discussion, however, was contradicted by the abundance of dread.

The second instance relating to bodily functions and motherhood was also connected with the birth process. This concerned the fact that the birth process is messy, involves blood and other bodily fluids, and is the primary period when transmission of HIV from mother to child occurs. It is a visceral process at the best of times, and one might expect the added complication of possible transmission to make it particularly frightening for HIV-positive mothers. In interviews, however, this was seldom discussed. When I asked the women what they were expecting (if they were pregnant) or what they had experienced (if they had already given birth), the responses were generally vague and non-committal. There were only two exceptions, both spontaneously raised in interviews. Both Ayanda and Lungile described seeing their blood on their babies during delivery. Ayanda tells how she thought about this during delivery and sat up in order to check whether her baby was safe from her blood, only to see her child covered with blood and coughing blood from her mouth.

You know the thing which makes me so scared, Carol? When I gave birth, I could see the blood <u>coming from</u>, you know, <u>coming from</u>, and that's how you pass it, coming from the mouth, the child was

coughing blood. I don't know whether all the babies do that during
the birth. Because I could see it. And the blood was coming out.

In this passage, Ayanda is trying to convey the horror of what she saw. There are
two points where she does not finish her train of thought (underlined above),
both concerning where the blood comes from. She then says the blood was
coming from her baby's mouth. What she cannot say aloud is that the blood
comes from her – it is her blood. At another point where she discusses this
experience, she similarly refers to 'the blood' or 'some blood'. It is clear from
her description, however, that she is looking for her blood, 'and that's how you
pass [HIV]'. Again, it is the confluence of the mother's body and the HIV-
positive body that threatens motherhood and life, as well as the confluence of
the mother's and the baby's blood that raises ambiguities that the mother has
infected the baby and that the baby has somehow infected the mother.

The third instance of the emergence of the infecting mother's body has
to do with the physical care of babies by mothers. Mandisa tells of a cut
on her hand:

Something cut me when I was at work and I had to put a bandage.
When I came back home, [my son] was sleeping and, you know, when
he wakes up, I have to play with him. And that cut in my hand started
bleeding, you know; I felt so terrible. I had to just leave him there on
the bed, you know, for me to just wipe off that blood, because I didn't
want my blood to touch him. You know, my gran, she just looked at
me and she didn't say anything and she just picked him up.

Mandisa describes being caught between different imperatives of
motherhood: to play with her son (the non-HIV variety) or to 'just leave
him there on the bed' in order to protect him from her blood (the HIV
variety). The HIV variety of motherhood wins out, but at cost to her sense
of self as a good mother. The motherly body cannot play with her son.
Tumi describes a similar occasion where she had a cut: 'I'm very afraid of

[my daughter] touching me, you know, being afraid that I might infect her, that I might infect my own family.' Her words vividly portray the fear of destroying those closest and most loved.

Why is this spoken about so seldom in interviews? A way into this issue is through its echoes in my own inabilities to think about infection. My supervisor was interested in talking about what it would mean for an HIV-positive mother to hold and care for her baby with the constant fear of possibly infecting the baby through such care and holding. Immersed in medical discourse as I was, I could not understand my supervisor's curiosity, because, of course, the mother was unlikely to infect her baby unless a significant amount of her blood managed to enter the inside of the baby's body. This was also not a major topic of discussion in interviews. Underneath my response, however, was my identification with the desperation with which respondents wanted to be good mothers, and I could not bear to think about everyday motherly care producing harm. I also missed the fact that the likelihood of such an event does not determine the level of fear; further, relative silence about an event does not indicate that there is no concern. What is striking about this silence is that fear of infection of one's baby permeates all the interviews, yet is seldom translated into everyday activities of the motherly body. This is a contradiction: of the ever presence of infection and then its sudden absence, and of the link between infection and motherhood, but not its link with the maternal body.

The very few points in interviews where the mother's body was directly invoked suggests that this silence does not simply indicate its unimportance, but rather that the mother's body is experienced as most frightening. With reference to her own body as a mother's body, the subjectivity of the HIV-positive mother appears to be overshadowed by infection. The bodily experience of motherhood can be difficult and terrifying, but it can also be creative and joyful. This analysis suggests that creativity and joy are censored and limited by HIV-infection. While this must be connected to very personal fears of destruction (of both self and other), these fears are amplified and given legitimacy by social discourses of HIV-positive motherhood. These can be more easily seen in the considerably more frequent reference to other HIV-positive mothers.

THE INFECTED MOTHER'S BODY MOST VISIBLE THROUGH STORIES OF OTHER MOTHERS

While there was silence regarding the self as infecting mother, stories abounded about other HIV-positive mothers. The mother's body itself was most frequently seen in the other, not the self. The ways in which other mothers were constructed suggests something about this particular kind of self-effacement. In the many stories about other mothers, there was a consistent split between good, idyllic mothers and bad, uncaring, irresponsible mothers, echoing similar splits in dominant constructions of motherhood. These splits (almost caricatures) were not only external, but were related to the self – the bodies of other mothers informed the subjectivity of interviewees.

The good mothers were commonly those found in the support group at the hospital. Most women commented on their admiration for these women, as well as the support they experienced from them. Ayanda, for example, relishes the company of these good mothers. It is not only their motherhood, however, that she values:

Oh, you feel great. You feel, ooh, we're in the same bus. You feel, you look at them, you try to look and see who's sick. You look at them; most of them, they're fine; and you look at the other ones as if, *ja*, that one, *ja*, uh-uh. You try to grab them and you feel like, um, you feel like you're in a family, you know. When you're together, but the thing is we don't stay together. I wish I was being with those ladies for the rest of my life.

Ayanda turns to these women as a point of comparison. They help her to evaluate herself as a 'good' mother, but also as an HIV-positive person. If they do not look sick, then she will be 'fine'. If she can emulate their mothering *as well as* their health, she can be part of the family. Constructions of good motherhood are thus intimately connected with constructions of good HIV-hood.

The power of these other mothers was consistently described as a sort of salvation. This may conceal the power of dominant discourses of HIV-positive motherhood. Anele's story throws the productive power of these discourses into relief. She was persuaded by the group to talk to me because she was considering giving her baby up for adoption. The other mothers were disapproving and seem to have put her under considerable pressure not only to talk to me, but, more concretely, to keep her baby. Anele was undecided about what to do. On the one hand, her repeated statements of love for her baby reinforced her desire to keep her baby, and she worried about how her baby would feel if adopted. She also worried that she would miss her baby. On the other hand, she was poor, her boyfriend had deserted her after she had disclosed her HIV status to him, she wanted her baby to grow up in a two-parent family and, most significantly, she could not bear the thought of either her baby being positive and dying or herself dying and leaving her baby. She repeated many times across the interview, 'I just can't leave my baby' – with reference to loss through death and not adoption – as well as, 'I just can't watch my baby die'. At one point, I asked her what she would choose if it were possible to ignore her baby's needs. After twice being unable to comprehend the question, she said,

Ignore? Truly speaking? I was gonna give my baby up for adoption. Because I wouldn't have to worry about raising a child, watching the child get sick and all this. And I was gonna get myself a better job than now, work for myself. So I have to stay at home now because I have a little one and I have to look after the baby for some few months and after that I have to go and look for a job. If I was to think for only me, really, I was gonna give my baby up. Because my other child is growing now. So I was gonna, I was really going to give my baby up.

Perhaps Anele can never fully occupy a position of motherhood that excludes her baby's needs, but the detail of her thought does emphasise that her words 'I just can't' represents a worry about her needs, a dread residing in her own identity as a mother. Her reasons for and against adoption also indicate how complex the decision is, for her baby as well as herself. This detail is provided in order to foreground the absolutism of discourses of motherhood she confronted in the support group. Towards the end of the interview, she says that she is now sure she will keep her baby:

> Before the support group, *ja*, I was not sure. Because it was like I was the only one who was going, because when, when, eh, that other counsellor told that, told them that, she asked me that can she tell them that I'm going to give my baby up and I said, '*ja*, you can tell them'. And she told them that I was going to give up my child for adoption, and everybody was, like, I didn't see even one person agreeing to that, you know; <u>everybody loved their</u> ... love, you know, I was like the only one who, who wanted to do <u>something that</u> .... I felt, I felt like I was a killer or something, you know. I felt like [pause] how can, how can I do that to my child, you know, because I know, I knew what they were thinking. That how can she do this to her baby, you know? How can she do that, how can she give the baby up just like that, you know?

Anele's decision is monitored through the eyes of other mothers. Her depiction graphically portrays normative discourses of motherhood at work: the only rule of motherhood is that sacrifice is made for one's baby. If this is not obeyed, then one is a bad mother. No other maternal response than selfless love can be tolerated. This overriding principle dissipates the complexities of her thoughts and feelings about what to do and replaces them with disapproving stares. The productive power of such discourses, to be taken on board as a way of monitoring one's self, is also clear. Confronting the unanimous response of women in the group, Anele *feels* like a killer and feels the shame of being constructed as a bad mother. She sees the point of view of selfless motherhood (which is an extreme position) and, positioning herself there, can acknowledge no other. This is reflected not only in her self-talk towards the end of the extract (imagining what 'they were thinking' and saying it to herself: 'how can she do this to her baby?'), but also in the two underlined segments. In both these cases, words fail her and she does not complete her sentence. In the first, 'everybody loved their', the missing word is 'baby' – the primary object of selfless motherhood. In the second, 'wanted to do something that' is left up to the imagination, but is clearly something bad that a mother *does* to her baby, and is followed immediately by a comment about the mother's destruction of her baby. This is the alternative position offered within the dominant discourse – that a mother's actions and desires can only be destructive if not in absolute service of the baby. The two unfinished sentences are in opposition to each other as the parameters of what is possible – love your baby or be a destructive mother. This is not to suggest that Anele should give her baby up for adoption, but rather that dominant discourses of motherhood construct what is legitimate, and, in this case, in simple and absolutist ways that deny aspects of her subjectivity in the process. This goes to the heart of the power of discourse over the mother's body, as well as her imperative to keep that body secondary to her baby. The extract illustrates its productive power through Anele enthusiastically taking on this discourse and then comparing and monitoring her subjectivity accordingly.

The group is enjoining Anele to position herself as a mother and to exclude her HIV-positive position from consideration. This was similarly expressed in frequent comments that women should not abort if they find they are HIV-positive because they are *primarily* a mother responsible for her baby's well-being and *secondarily* HIV-positive. The contradictions of this position are expressed by Hope. She says in her first interview that she had wanted to abort in order to protect her baby from infection, but had been diagnosed after her first trimester and was not legally allowed to undergo an abortion. In her second interview, she spontaneously says the opposite: 'it never came to my mind.' She then imagines other people looking at her and thinking that she is a bad person and mother because she is HIV-positive and has perhaps infected her baby. Nonetheless,

> I never thought of having an abortion, not even one day. Of course, I could see and imagine the difficulty that I am going to face, but I never thought of, you know, negative mind of having the abortion, or whatever.

The direct contradiction from one interview to the next illustrates possible contradictions between being a good mother by protecting the baby from infection and being a good mother in spite of infection (both options positing the overarching importance of the baby). Protecting the innocent baby may also hide the fantasy need to get rid of the dangerous baby, provoking guilt and denial.

When talking about other, idealised, HIV-positive mothers, the link to the self involves being primarily a mother. When talking about other denigrated HIV-positive mothers, however, 'bad motherhood' was consistently constructed as infecting motherhood, not motherhood despite infection. In the many stories of other bad HIV-positive mothers told in interviews, the tone was consistent: women described horror and anger at witnessing another HIV-positive woman breastfeeding her baby or becoming pregnant despite being aware of her status. The vehemence with which these stories were told exposes the power of dominant discourses of motherhood, as well as the horror of the HIV-positive body as either procreative (becoming pregnant) or carrying out maternal functions (breastfeeding). Even Lukanyo, who knew she was HIV-positive before becoming pregnant, describes her horror at the thought that somebody she knows might become pregnant again despite now being aware of her status. Typical of other stories, she stresses her disgust as she tells the story and also generalises in order to assert her moral position. She does this by referring to 'most women' who know they are HIV-positive:

[T]hey still come with a second pregnancy. And then the husband doesn't know, *né*, so they haven't told their husband from the first time that the first child is sick. Now they are coming again; they are pregnant again. So how do you cope with that? You see, they, they don't wanted to disclose and they don't wanted to protect themselves. … And how's [the mother] going to feel? Being a skeleton, bringing sickness for the baby. Even myself, I'll shudder when I see her [laughs].

Lukanyo is imagining women knowingly becoming pregnant and putting their babies at risk. Her image, typically, is abject (Kristeva, 1982); it evokes a shudder and the image of a skeleton. She constructs these women as not wanting to protect themselves or their babies, and therefore as deserving of their feelings of wretchedness and the observer's disgust and scorn. What she is describing is the pinnacle of bad motherhood because of its *infectious* nature (in both the procreative and the viral sense). No reference is made to the contradiction that she knowingly became pregnant.

This example also illustrates the importance of these stories in providing women with objects against which to construct themselves as mothers and stories through which the women could express their fear of their badness as mothers in disguised ways. Lukanyo is able to construct herself in opposition to 'most women' – as a good mother and as able to recognise the badness of others – as well as to distance herself from her own fear of having infected her baby that emerges at other points in the interview. This is most strikingly accomplished in her shudder and her laugh, which make these bad mothers different from 'even myself'.

One other example will be given to illustrate the construction of the self in opposition to bad mothers, and the way in which this offers the opportunity to shift guilt away from the self. In this example, Phindiwe is expressing her relief that her baby has not been sick, and her hope that this indicates that he is negative. She then says:

Phindiwe: He's just fine. You know, some mothers, they say their babies, like, when you find out you're HIV, they want to breastfeed the child. Oh, some they breastfeed, the mothers knowing that they are HIV-positive.

CL: What do you think that's about for them?

Phindiwe: Maybe they're, they don't, they just want their baby to go with them.

CL: They don't want to leave their baby behind. And for you?

Phindiwe: I won't breastfeed. A baby's an angel; you don't have to put your sins on the baby.

For Phindiwe, it is self-evident why these mothers are bad. She does not give a reason, merely repeating their bad action: 'they breastfeed.' When prompted to wonder why, she imagines them thinking about their own maternal desires: 'they just want their baby to go with them.' Ironically, this statement was formulated by a number of women in interviews in order to express motherhood from their own point of view in terms of the pain of having to leave their babies. Here, however, the statement is connected clearly to infection and constructs 'bad' mothers as selfish and destructive. By constructing herself in opposition to these bad mothers, Phindiwe clearly splits selfishness and destructiveness away from herself. However, her explanation for not breastfeeding, for not being like the bad women – 'you don't have to put your sins on the baby' – resonates with more close-to-home fears she expresses at other points. Phindiwe is scared that she has done exactly this. She describes, for example, feeling like a 'bad mother' for possibly infecting her child.[1] Perhaps her construction of other mothers as bad allows her not only to construct herself in opposition as good, but also to project some of her own feelings of badness onto them and thereby process them in ways that do not threaten her wish to be a good mother.

1 This was discussed before she discovered that her son was in fact HIV-negative.

Whether idealised or denigrated, then, maternal bodies are more visible in interviews through other mothers than through the bodies of the women themselves. Subjectivities of motherhood are constructed by these stories in relation to the importance of the mother's versus the baby's perspective, as well as to the relative importance of motherhood versus infection. This illustrates the dynamic tension between being a mother to a baby and being a mother oneself, as well as the impossibility of positioning oneself either within or in opposition to dominant discourses of HIV and motherhood. Unsurprisingly, perhaps, the final place where the mother's body was directly evoked is in the intersection of mother, baby and infection.

THE BABY'S STATUS CHANGING THE MOTHER'S BODY

The only other points where the mother's body was directly evoked occurred where women contemplated their babies' status. In the process of evaluating their babies' bodies, their own bodies became foregrounded not only as HIV-positive, but as maternal. Contemplation of the baby's status allows space not only for the mother's body to become more visible, but also for the mother's own subjectivity. Through the primary position of the baby in these moments, mothers could voice something that was just for them as mothers.

Lukanyo, for example, imagines herself becoming a mother and feels that she will gain weight through the happiness of motherhood – that the existence of her baby will make her healthy. In two different interviews she refers to the interchangeability of the mother's body with the baby's body:

[Imagining her baby being born:] I think I will gain, I will even gain more weight, maybe because I will always, you know, [be] smiling; they say the heart it's always happy, you gain more weight, gain more weight, because you're coming more happier. I think I will be more happier than before.

[After her baby's birth:] Now I'm a mother. I'm still fine; I don't look sick. The baby, it doesn't look sick; it looks fat, more fatter. So, I, that was the thing that, that was one of my wishes, was to be a mother. And then, and I was trying to show the people that to have a disease doesn't mean that it's the end of the world. You can have some other things that you want.

While pregnant, Lukanyo imagines her body becoming healthy through the happiness that her child will bring her. The joy of motherhood allows the maternal body to overcome the HIV-positive body. When her baby is born, she scans her child's body and sees signs of her own health within it. Here, the fantasy is that the baby will cure rather than infect. This very personal observation and desire is linked to the way in which 'the people' see her (people living in her area often gossip about her HIV status). Looking at herself through her baby allows her to feel healthy. It offers her a point of resistance against prejudice and also against the feeling that desire (the 'things that you want') has not been utterly destroyed and that she can have motherhood for herself. This position, in which she approaches motherhood through her own desires, is, of course, in jeopardy, contradicted at other points in interviews by her fears that her baby will be sick and that she is culpable. Nonetheless, it is a position in which she can reframe herself through the identity of motherhood and the interconnection between herself and her baby.

At times, then, the baby (and therefore motherhood) was a saviour. For Lukanyo, salvation comes with the fact of motherhood, but this is contingent on the health of her baby. This was often the case. For example, Ayanda feels that 'if I hear my baby is negative, that will, it will boost my immune [system] as well'. Women would often say that if their babies were negative, they (the women) would not only become healthier, but would in fact be cured. Lesedi acknowledges that her own cure through her baby's salvation is a fantasy, but in its promise, this does not matter to her. She imagines hearing that her baby is negative and imagines forcing a reversal of her own status:

Ja, I will be happy if it's just, if she, if she's negative, you know. Maybe I'll even forget that; I will thought that the doctors make a mistake. I'll take it that, I'll make it in my mind that I tested negative. They made a mistake that I'm positive. The baby's negative, so I'm also negative. Knowing that I'm not.

If Lesedi's baby is safe, Lesedi can indulge the fantasy that she is safe because of the relief she will feel: 'The baby's negative so I'm also negative.' The baby's body is not the mother's body, but the mother's body is at least potentially also the baby's body.

Because this is a realm of opposites and reversals, however, many women also imagined hearing that their babies were positive and imagined their (maternal) bodies being destroyed as a result. Some women imagined that the news would kill them, make them sick or increase their viral load. When Zinzi, for example, hopes that her baby will be negative and says, 'maybe I will die, if they tell me that he is positive', her earnest tone suggests that she does not believe that her maternal body will survive. Many women imagined negative bodily consequences for themselves as a result of the shock of discovering that they had infected their babies, implying that the mother's body cannot and should not survive – that it should be punished for infecting the baby's body or that the baby has succeeded in destroying the mother. From the perspective of the baby, the maternal body is imagined to reflect the guilt of being a bad mother. Khanya's comment illustrates that this dimension also has its reverse: the mother's body is secondary, but also primary:

[I]f the baby's positive obviously, whatever pains she feels, I'm going to feel the same pains, because, knowing that I'm HIV-positive, I'm going to have that mind that something like this is going to happen to me, as well some other time.

Imagining that her baby is HIV-positive, she imagines guilt and reflects this in the parallel between her baby's pains and her own. Observing a sick baby does not only evoke the guilt of being an infecting mother, but also the similarity between mother and baby. 'Something like this is going to happen to me as well': the mother's body will also become sick. It is not only guilt that connects mother and baby, but also experience.

The baby could therefore save the mother's body or condemn it – either bring a miracle or an apocalypse; either confirm women as good mothers or confirm their guilt and badness; either bring salvation or cause destruction. The mother's body exists most strongly as a space on which punishment or reprieve could be written, depending entirely on what they had done to their babies, which, in fantasy, may equate to what their babies had done to them.

CONCLUSION

The maternal body is symbolic of creativity – by its ability to grow and change in order to create life and then by its presence in making meaning of motherhood. Without the addition of HIV, the maternal body can be equally symbolic of destructiveness and is therefore symbolically powerful. HIV within the maternal body is also both creative and destructive. When the maternal body entered interviews, surreptitiously or indirectly, this power of simultaneous creativity and destructiveness was present, whether in the form of procreation versus murder, mother destroying baby or baby destroying mother, idealisation versus denigration, or salvation versus condemnation. These poles were often kept as separate as the good and bad mothers in the social world. Mothers visited their own bodies, but also saw themselves through other (both good and bad) mothers, as well as through the meaning that their bodies were given through the meanings of the bodies of their babies. The ways in which women watched maternal bodies in this chapter suggest processes of self-surveillance in which social anxieties about good versus bad mothers become turned on the self. The power of discourses of motherhood then becomes an internally powerful process of observation and correction, as if keeping badness in check. Examination of the mother's body goes only part of the way towards bringing the mother's subjectivity into the foreground, because it is largely a body of absence. Where it is most present, it is brought to the foreground by the existence of infection or by concern for the baby. This chapter has suggested that constructions of the maternal body allow the exploration of a space within subjectivity that can be occupied from the mother's perspective. Processes of surveillance of the maternal body help to make the secondary nature of maternity more visible, but the maternal body also undermines dominant discourses of motherhood, because it refuses to be ignored. Maternal bodies would not be denied. Silent, perhaps, but not invisible; seen more easily through others than through the self, but not entirely split; destructive, but also creative; and that which is a mother's own.

8. Thula Mama

'*Thula mama*': 'hush, mother'. The title of this chapter represents an inversion of words said by mothers to babies over countless generations, words inspiring many South African lullabies and the famous 'hush little baby, don't you cry', originating in Africa and sung by mothers to their children around the world. It has been chosen for the title of this chapter precisely because of its inversion of the subject: the words are surprising because the commonly received idiom is '*thula baba*'. The mother is expected to be the speaker of these words, but not their subject. This chapter takes as its focus the mother's subjectivity from the position of speaking subject. Within this, there is another reason for the title being chosen: 'Hush little baby, don't you cry' implies the centrality of the baby and his/her needs and emotions, and thereby the unimportance of the mother's needs and emotions. It is immediately followed, however, by 'mama's gonna sing you a lullaby'. The lullaby encapsulates one of the central paradoxes of motherhood: in the very moment that the mother is effaced, her voice and her words are there to comfort and also to create. The lullaby creates comfort and beauty for both the baby and the mother, because it belongs to the mother, given to her by her mother. Perhaps lullabies are the beginnings of women's writing. Mama is speaking of *her* love for her baby as well as of *her* fears. By stepping into the perspective of her baby, she is most able to be a mother herself.

While acknowledging that the subjectivity of the mother can never be separated from concern for her baby, this chapter nonetheless takes as its focus '*thula mama*' and not '*thula baba*'. The chapter seeks the HIV-positive mother's identity *as a mother* and from the mother's point of view – the moments in interviews when women spoke about what it meant for them to be mothers, sometimes selfishly, often apologetically, anxiously, sometimes almost accidentally. The analysis will suggest that, quite contrary to the majority of literature on motherhood and on HIV-positive mothers, as well as to cultural discourses concerning the passivity and relative unimportance of the experience of motherhood *for the mother*, women did occupy positions in which the primary subject was herself, not another. Perhaps because of the power of discourses of motherhood, this subject position was often taken up only in brief moments. This chapter often considers not just repetitions, but also exceptions and absences in the interview material related to the ways in which the women constructed themselves as HIV-positive mothers. It will be suggested that the mother's position is one of absence, hovering in the margins of what is allowable to say, but that it is also an identity of excess – excess of meaning; excess of emotion – and is therefore simultaneously excluded from dominant discourses and uncontainable by discourse.

This simultaneous absence and excess of meaning is implied in the words '*thula mama*'. The words could mean 'silence, mother', implicating the silencing of mothers' experiences by social discourses of motherhood and the latter's overarching emphasis on the well-being of the baby. It could also mean 'don't worry, mother' – indicating a need to soothe the mother's pain, and that the mother *has* pain separate to that of her baby or her concern for her baby. An alternative possible meaning is, 'be still mother; go to sleep', evoking in the context of the lullaby a 'little sleep', but, in the context of HIV, the much bigger sleep of death. Where the literature on HIV-positive motherhood is concerned about harm or death to the baby, the mothers interviewed were also concerned about their own deaths and about the loss *to themselves* of motherhood. This meaning reminds one of the proximity of HIV-positive motherhood to life and to death. Finally, because '*thula mama*' is appropriated from the beauty of mothers singing lullabies, it is also potentially a refusal to be silenced and a celebration of the joys of being a mother. It therefore also has connotations of 'sing your heart out; sing your joy and love'.

These echoes – of the silencing of the speaking mother within discourse and of the centrality of pain, death and joy to the subjectivity of HIV-positive motherhood – are central to the analysis. The chapter, in an attempt to explore these meanings from the position of motherhood, will suggest that, while they cannot be reconciled with one another, they can also not be disentangled from one another. Further, it will be argued that occupying a speaking position as a mother involves occupying tensions between profound opposites, e.g. between love and hate, tragedy and joy, and life and death. In relation to the baby, there is one subject: the good and innocent baby. From the perspective of the mother herself, however, mother and baby are both subject and object and are also potentially interchangeable: the infecting mother with the infecting baby, the healthy baby with the healthy mother, the baby's loss with the mother's loss.

Exploration of where and how the mother's voice exists also entails exploration of the primacy of the baby; in searching for the active position of motherhood, the secondary position cannot be separated out. It will be suggested that the baby is discursively primary, although the mother is secondary; that the position of the active mother herself is present if not dominant; but that their mutual exclusivity implied by dominant discourses of motherhood (e.g. good, selfless mother versus bad, selfish mother) cannot account for the interconnectedness of subjectivities of motherhood.

Reflecting on the previous chapter, the mother's body suggests all the connotations of '*thula mama*'. Perhaps the most dominant remains 'be quiet – don't speak about yourself as a mother', but this exists in dynamic tension with other possible meanings. Talk about maternal bodies also suggests the tension between the need to soothe the pain of being an HIV-positive mother and the joys of motherhood reflected back at one through one's baby. Around the perimeters of all these meanings is also the implication that the mother will 'go to sleep' and leave her baby through death. This dynamic interplay of meanings of motherhood remains central in this chapter, with its focus on what the women said about motherhood. Ironically, given the imperative of dominant discourse to 'be quiet – don't speak about yourself as a mother', the mother as primary subject was most easily visible, if not most frequently expressed, through what the women said about their desires and fears as mothers.

The majority of the discussion on motherhood was undertaken from the perspective of the baby. Answers to direct questions about the experience of motherhood often came across as unidimensional, vague and unelaborated. Petunia's answer is illustrative: 'A mother is a woman with a baby. When you have a baby, you have to be a mother.' Her statement almost reflects a lack of meaning, as if motherhood means nothing to her beyond her responsibility for her baby. The women frequently discussed motherhood in terms of the all-importance of their babies. Leleti's reflection on motherhood is illustrative:

> *Leleti:* [W]hen you're a mother, you must be strong. Then, don't say, don't think about people, what people are going to say and all that, just think about you and your baby .... Like, if your baby's sick, you don't have to take anything personally. You know, like, that God doesn't love you and all that; you must be strong. Being a mother is very important ....
>
> *CL:* In what ways do you think you are a good mother and in what ways do you think you are a bad mother?
>
> *Leleti:* To be a good mother, it's things like taking care of the baby and making the baby my first priority. If I've got money, I can't

even buy anything for myself; I just think about the baby, buy milk and all those things .... So being a bad mother, just to be HIV, and I mustn't, like, die.

Leleti describes steeling herself against herself – not 'tak[ing] anything personally' – by focusing completely on her baby's needs and 'making the baby my first priority'. Motherhood is defined as an excising of her own needs and emotions for the good of her baby and occurs within a socioeconomic context of limited resources. Being a good mother means subsuming herself: her own desire to be a good mother means foregoing her own desires. Leleti echoes the overarching desire of women in this study to be good mothers, almost as if to preserve this ultimately good aspect of their lives from anything bad.

Her response to being a 'bad' mother – 'to be HIV, and I mustn't, like, die' – is also typical and suggests the foe that the 'good' mother is up against: her HIV status dominates her definition of bad motherhood. This interview question about good and bad aspects of motherhood, prompted by Parker's (1995) exploration of the ambivalence of motherhood, was routinely answered with reference to the 'good' focus on baby rather than self and to the 'bad' existence of the virus, either through its threat of infecting the baby or through the death of the mother, as well as the woman. Notably, the dominant alternative answer to the good versus bad parts of motherhood was to ignore or deny the possibility of being a bad mother at all. Lungile, for example, simply answers, 'I am a good mother'. Thandiwe, who asks for the question to be repeated three times, eventually says:

Hey, I don't imagine myself to be a bad mother; I don't I tell you. I always wanted to be a good mother .... So I don't see myself as a bad mother, you see? ... So I'm trying all the time that I'm being a good mother ... I'm trying by all means to make [my son] happy all the time, *ja*. So I don't see myself as a bad mother, *ja*; I always dreamed of being a good mother, to be a good example to them.

It is not an option for Thandiwe to in any way imagine herself to be a bad mother. This is poignantly contradicted in her next interview, where she describes being wracked with guilt about being a bad mother, because of her fear that 'maybe I've done a bad thing to my baby'. While Thandiwe's response enforces the all-importance of the baby ('I'm trying by all means to make [my son] happy all the time'), however, she is also inhabiting motherhood through her own needs: she wants to be a good mother because it means a great deal to her. While recognising the dominance of discourses of the facelessness and selflessness of motherhood, the mothers also resisted this through voicing their joys and fears, their hopes and desires for themselves as mothers, not only for their babies.

When the women did speak from this location, there was typically an expression of extremes of emotion characterised by tensions between tragedy and joy. In order to introduce these conflicts, three case studies will be presented. The first two have been chosen because the mothers expressed, largely through fantasy, more forbidden aspects of motherhood than were present in other interviews, but much more surreptitiously voiced. The third case study focuses on the multiplicity of motherhood through the story of one particular woman. The cases will help contextualise the primacy of motherhood from the mother's perspective in the stories and voices of individual women and in the social and emotional complexities of being an HIV-positive mother. The case studies will lead into a discussion of the ways in which tensions between opposites, notably tragedy and joy, become crucial points of negotiation in the business of constructing motherhood.

NOMBEKO: LOVE AND HATE

Nombeko was one of the few women to explicitly describe anger towards her baby, who, she felt in fantasy, had given her HIV. Nombeko's story was introduced in chapter 3. Here, the issue of maternal ambivalence, and anger and fear in particular, will be explored in more detail.

The relative absence of anger from the position of the mother herself links to a silence across interviews that Nombeko contravened. She considers the medical treatment that she receives compared to her baby:

> Sometimes I feel sick. I feel sick and the thing is the government doesn't know about my status; it's just [the hospital], and [the hospital] is more concerned about my baby. About me, they don't want to know. And the thing is that makes me, my life, too much difficult.

Nombeko is referring to the bias that prioritises the baby, but ignores the mother – '[a]bout me, they don't want to know'. Not only was this bias towards treating the child seldom discussed across interviews, but when it was, it was done with remarkably little anger. Nombeko was one of the few exceptions. It seemed that women were so grateful to get something for their babies, particularly when they knew many women were not, that they could not express anger about the fact that their babies were getting something that they should have been getting too. The silence is noteworthy because lack of treatment for mothers represents one of the most material ways in which the position of motherhood as secondary and less important is legitimised. The implication is that babies need protection, but mothers do not. Anger towards the government was notably absent; so too was anger towards the baby.

Given the centrality of maternal hate (Long, 2007; Winnicott, 1987) and maternal ambivalence (Parker, 1995) – i.e. the coexistence of love and hate – to motherhood, and the simultaneity with which the women in this study discovered they were pregnant and HIV-positive, one would perhaps expect them to have mixed feelings towards their babies. This was surprisingly absent from interviews, with women clearly and repeatedly expressing only very positive sentiments about their children. Occasionally, some women would mention a different kind of feeling, but this remained largely unelaborated. Ayanda, for example, once referred to her 'disaster baby', meaning that her baby had brought disaster to her, but this remained unexplored and contradicted by repeated positive statements about her baby. Lesedi described hating her baby for leading her to discover that she was HIV-positive – but only in the past tense. She explained that since she had seen other HIV-positive mothers loving their babies, she had 'accepted', and the hatred had completely dissipated. Hlengiwe briefly said that since she heard she was HIV-positive, 'I'm starting to resent, somewhere, somehow, my baby … I feel like I'm not going to love my baby like I'm supposed to'. In all of these statements, a different kind of feeling was stated and then left unelaborated, not to be returned to again.

Nombeko also spoke fluently about her love for her baby. Anything else was mentioned briefly, and in the past tense. She described, for example, hitting her stomach with her fist when she was pregnant – 'I was so angry to be pregnant' – and hating her baby for infecting her, because at the time she needed to 'transfer blame' for being HIV-positive. She also described an ongoing process of being too scared to love her baby, in case he was only 'borrowed' to her. In this way, she expressed her fear of both hating too much *and* loving too much. Nombeko was scared that her hatred would destroy her love, but could, in retrospect, accept the existence of both her hatred and, retrospectively and presently, her love. Perhaps fear of the fantasised infecting baby and fear of having infected her baby, both centrally concerned with attacks on and the destructiveness of one's maternal self, made the direct expression of anger too dangerous.

Nombeko was one of the few women to express ambivalence directly; she also told a story that may help to explain the lack of expressed ambivalence in interviews. The story arose at a point where she is wondering what she will do if her baby is HIV-positive:

Nombeko: [T]here was a lady, she was positive, she get pregnant and she have a positive baby, you know. She just take a pillow and put it on top of the baby and said, 'I don't want to look at my baby suffering'. You know? You feel, if I'm going to be stressed because of my baby, you know, maybe my baby is going to die, and then, after, it's going to be me. So I want to be relieved, like I was, I was so relieved. I even told my mother, you know [pause].

CL: So that lady who put a pillow over her baby; you can understand?

Nombeko: Yes, I can understand and I can; I told my mother I can do that too. The way I am, I can do that, because looking at your baby suffering is like punishing him or her, you know. That lady wasn't supposed to be, she wasn't locked up. No. She told them that 'I didn't want to see my baby suffering'. You know, this disease can do such horrible things to babies like this one, *ja*.

It should be stressed that, as Nombeko related this story, there was no sense that she would actually kill her baby, but rather that she was indulging in a fantasy that allowed her to express forbidden emotions through the 'legitimate' story of a woman who loved her baby and whom nobody blamed for what she had done: 'she wasn't locked up' (this element of the story further suggests fantasy is at play: in real life, the police would not be understanding). Through this story, she can imagine destroying her baby and thereby express her anger towards her baby and fear of her own destructiveness and defend herself against the fear that her baby may destroy her. The story also allows her a 'solution' to her guilt that leaves her blameless and loving, as well as offering her a defence against the link between her baby's death and her own ('maybe my baby is going to die, and then, after, it's going to be me'). The power of the story also throws the general absence of any direct expression of ambivalence into relief. In a terrain of motherhood so beset with possibilities for destruction, why is maternal ambivalence so unseen?

Perhaps this question cannot be answered, but an exploration of the dominant possibilities open to HIV-positive mothers may provide some hypotheses. Perhaps because of the very public associations between HIV and destruction, maternal ambivalence becomes particularly dangerous –

to the point that *any* expression of anger from the position of mother risks opening the door for devastating destructiveness to enter. This links with the interconnectedness of HIV and motherhood. Maternal ambivalence was exclusively connected to HIV, and projections of destructiveness onto the baby linked concretely to fantasies of infection. All other normal and common expressions of ambivalence (Parker, 1995) were absent. It is suggested that this is not only because HIV holds such overwhelming personal meaning, but also because of the social constructions of HIV-positive motherhood as aberrant, destructive and forbidden. Further, the expression of ambivalence is perhaps silenced by positions available within dominant discourse. Maternal ambivalence belongs squarely to the mother as subject, and potentially contradicts the selflessness expected by dominant discourses of motherhood, in which the baby is the only subject.

NONYAMEKO: LIFE AND DEATH

Nonyameko was diagnosed HIV-positive (with two separate tests) when she was three months pregnant. We met for the first time when her daughter was three months old, and conducted four interviews over a period of five months. She disclosed her status to her husband almost immediately, and they jointly decided not to tell friends or family for fear of stigmatisation. She now suspects that she contracted HIV from her previous fiancée, with whom she had a baby who suddenly and inexplicably became sick and died. After learning of her diagnosis, she began to suspect that the baby died of AIDS-related illness. She then met and married her current husband. She was pleased when she fell pregnant, as they had been trying to conceive for some time.

In our first interview, Nonyameko was matter-of-fact about her diagnosis, repeating, 'what can you do? There is nothing that I can do'. She was expecting results for her husband and baby, and we arranged to meet after these results had been received. Like other women, she wished for a cure, but knew that there was no cure at present.

This took a dramatic turn when we met for a second interview. Nonyameko told me that her husband and baby were negative, and that blood tests had revealed that she was also negative and had been 'cured'. She believed that she had been HIV-positive, but was cured because of the medication that she had received to induce labour. At that point, I knew that a sudden negative result was extremely unlikely, but walked away from the interview feeling angry that the doctors had falsely diagnosed her (in the absence of any anger from her in this regard) and guilty for thinking that she might be fantasising a negative result.

In our third interview, she told me the story again as if I had never heard it before and as if she had just discovered that she was negative. Her narrative was more elaborated this time, including, for example, saying that she had tested negative three times and giving detailed descriptions of the doctors' shock at her negative diagnosis and their desire to do 'experiments' on her because they thought they might be able to find a cure for other women. She wanted me to speak to the doctors, and I was relieved to gain permission to do this, because I was beginning to suspect from her elaborated tale that there was at least an element of fantasy at play.

The hospital confirmed that no blood tests (HIV or otherwise) had been recently conducted on her. This meant that she had not physically given blood at any point during the previous months. There was no record of a reversed diagnosis. Her HIV-positive status was then confirmed by a viral load test,[1] and she was given this result just before our final interview. Nonyameko was disappointed with the result. She did not offer an explanation about how the misunderstanding had occurred, but said: 'It's done, there's nothing, need to accept it, but for me it's, you know, I'll be putting myself as negative.' Her baby's negative result was confirmed.

Although this is a story about Nonyameko's status as an HIV-positive *person*, her fantasy of cure is centrally connected to her position as a *mother*

---

1   An HIV test measures antibodies and is thus less accurate than the viral load test, which measures the virus itself.

in two important ways. Firstly, the best explanation for what happened, based on the way in which she told her story, is that she had taken her baby to give blood on three occasions and, while she herself had not physically given blood, had somehow linked her baby's tests with her own. Her description of the tests that she took and the point when she was told she was negative corresponds exactly with her baby's tests and subsequent negative result. This suggests that her fantasy was catalysed by an identity of motherhood in which news of her baby's negative status was immediately related to herself. If her baby is negative, her position as secondary to her baby is safer, but her position as a mother herself remains unaltered. Given the potential for interchangeability between mother and baby, Nonyameko heard salvation for her baby as salvation for herself as well. Her baby was not destructive and would not be destroyed by her, and so her own destructive HIV parts were literally removed.

This highlights the link between motherhood and HIV. In fact, the first time she mentions 'cure' in her first interview is in response to a question about her experience of motherhood:

The best part, I enjoy my baby very much. There's nothing I can do. Maybe they will find out there's a cure for it. I can have another one. A little boy. Just that maybe they must find a cure but [pause].

Nonyameko contemplates her experience of motherhood and immediately shifts to acknowledging the presence of HIV in this identity. At this point, she imagines a cure for both herself and her baby. Her fantasy of being cured herself arises when she finds that her baby is negative. In this first mention, Nonyameko makes reference to the second important aspect that connects her story of cure to identities of motherhood. If she can be cured, 'I can have another [baby]'. If she is HIV-positive, the procreative aspect of motherhood for herself is taken away because of the risk of infecting another baby. The possibility of procreation is intimately woven into the process of her interviews. In her first interview, where she is HIV-positive, she wishes for another baby, but only if there is a cure for HIV. In her second and third interviews, where she believes herself to be cured, she repeatedly describes conversations in which either her husband or her doctors urge her to have another baby. She describes steadfastly refusing until she is sure of her negative diagnosis, and stresses that she is continuing to use condoms despite being cured, just in case. Her description of the doctors' eagerness for her to procreate (an unlikely medical stance) suggests that the fantasy of having another child is hers. This wish gains another dimension when she stresses that, in addition to their daughter, her husband wants her to have a son to replace the son that she previously lost. If she does not have any more children, she will never again be a mother to a son. It is only at the end of our final interview, once she again believed herself to be HIV-positive, that she reframes the desire for another baby as her own:

> I was thinking about maybe another baby. They were saying, the dad, not to sleep with him. They take his sperm, they inject it, whatever, and then you can be pregnant. Now I don't know, *ja*; maybe I'll ask Dr S. Maybe we can do that. But me, I'm HIV-positive. Now to do it again, I will get more sensitive; you know what I mean? So that's the way it is; one baby, it's okay.

It becomes clear at this point that although Nonyameko has hitherto been insisting that other people (and not herself) want her to procreate, she has thought in detail about having another baby. The significance of HIV in the context of motherhood is that she feels that the option of procreation has been denied her. Many women were adamant about not having another baby and disgusted with women who did; Nonyameko's story suggests that the desire to have another baby – a desire belonging to the mother herself – is one that does not simply disappear with the advent of HIV. Although Nonyameko's is an extreme story, it illustrates the very complex relationship between life and death, as well as between mother and baby.

JOYCE: ALONE IN CONTEXT

Joyce's story illustrates the dynamic tension between different fears and desires, as well as the interrelationships between a mother of a baby and a mother from her own perspective. Her story also allows us to consider motherhood intergenerationally and in context. Every woman's story was unusual in some way; Joyce's stood out because her mother had died of AIDS a few years previously. This was the first thing she told me, and the consequences of this story, which was as important to her as the story of being HIV-positive herself, unfolded gradually during her interview. Joyce was at school when her mother became sick. As the firstborn, she had to leave school in order to nurse her mother through the final stages of the disease and to look after her siblings. She had to send her first child, a daughter, to live with her mother-in-law, because her time was taken up caring for her mother. Her daughter remained there after her mother died. Her father then rejected her, but not her siblings, and her siblings followed suit. As a result, she was ostracised from the family. She was then diagnosed HIV-positive when she was three months pregnant with her second child.

One would expect Joyce's story to underline intergenerational and contextual aspects of motherhood. She felt that she knew she was a good mother, because 'I saw it with my mother', but she also feared becoming sick, because she had seen that with her mother too. In a way, she knew more than the other women interviewed about HIV-positive motherhood, because she was both an HIV-positive mother and the daughter of an HIV-positive mother. Further, the fact that her family story was so important to her tempts one to imagine the importance of family to the experience of motherhood.

On the other hand, however, the story of her broader family context was kept remarkably separate from her story of motherhood. Her experience, particularly with her mother and father, resonated with issues of motherhood, but, like almost all the women interviewed, she constructed motherhood as an individual affair. In stark contrast to (often romanticised) notions of the 'extended family', the women invariably constructed motherhood as their role alone, expressing protectiveness over this role, but also isolation as a result. In Joyce's case, this was clearest in her description of motherhood as the most important identity in her life. She stressed that her love for her children was what kept her strong and that she wanted to do everything possible for her children: 'I want to be here for my babies.' When talking about motherhood, nobody else had a part to play. Also kept separate from these conversations was the fact that she had had to give up daily care of her older daughter because she was living with her paternal grandparents. This is a common, but historically recent cultural practice, having more to do with urbanisation and the urban–rural divide than with expectations of the caring function of the extended family. She hated being far away from her daughter and sadly related that her daughter would only call her 'mom' when they were alone together. She constructed motherhood as belonging only to her, but contextually did not have access to being that kind of mother to her older child.

Joyce's story illustrates the individuality of motherhood that pervaded interviews, while at the same time raising questions about the role of the extended family. A common assumption made regarding HIV in the context of the African family is that the extended family network is a protective factor, and this assumption often runs towards the more extreme version that one does not need to be concerned about 'black people', because their kinship networks will take care of everything. Perhaps the notion of the protective extended family has always been a myth, particularly because it does not account for the dynamics within families and thereby presupposes a complete and unrealistic entity. With the increase of Westernisation and the erosion of families by urbanisation (Guy, 1990) and by HIV (Walker, Reid & Cornell, 2004), the extended family becomes even more elusive. This was illustrated in the stories of many women; Joyce's illustrates the loss of family members to HIV, the loss of family through conflicts unrelated to HIV, and the conflict between her individualised aspirations of motherhood and her distance from her older child. Individualising discourses of motherhood, together with little practical recourse to the myth of the extended family, leave her with an abiding desire to be with family and to be the only mother to her children – to have this identity all to herself – within a context in which family ties are tenuous and motherhood indirect.

TRAGEDY AND JOY

Almost all the women identified motherhood as their primary identity of joy and as the one part of their lives where they could have something special purely for themselves. Although the secondary nature of the mother remains dominant in musings on motherhood, the primacy of identities of motherhood is present and articulated. Women did want something just for themselves as mothers; they expressed desires and fears that were theirs alone. Mothers became the subjects of motherhood fleetingly, but not quietly. The moments when women spoke about experiences of motherhood from their own perspective (and here it is important for the analysis to pay attention to the personal pronoun 'me') were frequently moments of extreme emotion and expressions of tragedy or joy.

This tragedy or joy was described as belonging to the mother, not only to the baby. Neo encapsulates her own pleasure in being a mother:

> It's like a dream come true, you know, because watching your kids every day, growing, it's a very nice thing, you know. I enjoy it, even if she's six weeks, you know. At some points she, she hears you, you know, turning her head, or just trying to talk, you know. It's like a dream come true, you know? ... Mm, it's very, very nice.

This 'dream come true' is for Neo – it belongs to her. Her enjoyment is her own and is reinforced when her baby 'turn[s] her head' towards her and recognises her as her mother. Her joy is her own and her identity is seen. This is, of course, tinged for Neo by her fear of dying and her determination to be a good mother to her children: 'I must have strength and power to live for my kids, you know'; but does not obliterate her joy.

The tragedy of death was foremost for many women, finding expression in sadness about babies losing a mother, but also in the personal loss to mothers of having to leave their babies behind when they died. Hlengiwe tearfully recounts how the joys of motherhood are edged with the helplessness of not being able to save her baby, but also with the painful loss of her baby through her own death:

Being a mom, it's a nice experience, but knowing that you are HIV-positive changes everything again. Because you have to think, 'I'm positive; what about my baby? What about me?' Okay, at the clinic they can save the baby, but what about me, the mother? I cannot save the baby. I die earlier, then my baby is going to suffer … I know I love my baby, but maybe at the end of the day I'm going to lose him or her, so it's very difficult.

Hlengiwe wants to be able to save her baby herself; she does not want to be the passive bystander. Her helplessness and, perhaps, her feeling of being robbed of one of the joys of motherhood lead her to imagine a more final situation where she will be unable to help her baby. Of course, the pain she feels is the pain of her baby's loss, but it is also palpably her own. It is not just that her baby is going to lose her, but that *she* is going to lose her baby: 'I'm going to lose.' Each loss, from its different perspective, is important. This led many of the women to wish to live at least long enough to see their babies grow bigger, so that their babies could have as much of them as possible, but also so that they themselves could experience motherhood for as long as possible and so that their babies could remember them – that their identities as mothers would last beyond death. The joy of being known as a mother is necessary in the face of the tragedy of being lost. In Lungile's words, 'I feel free because, like, just, he knows me'. If her baby knows her, her identity is not lost.

From the mother's perspective, tragedy resides not only in the loss to herself of her children, but also in the loss of motherhood through death. Women did not want to have to give up being mothers. Thandiwe illustrates this after she distances herself from her fears about her baby's status: 'I don't think about that; I don't have that on my mind; I don't want it. I just see him as a happy child.' Perhaps because she has symbolically taken care of her baby, at least for the moment, she then moves from her baby's well-being to her own:

[T]he only thing, the only person that I think about all the time, it's me. Mm, I've got that worry, mm, me. I just wonder, how long will I live, you know? How much time God will give me, to see him grow? [*In another interview:*] And that's the only thing that is stressing me, that I don't know how long I'm going to spend time with my baby.

Thandiwe's concern for herself is not only about dying, but specifically about losing her identity of motherhood: how much time will *she* have to be a mother. She is concerned about loss of her own maternal gaze ('me to see him grow'). Her concern about herself as a mother is interlinked with her concern about her baby, but it nonetheless exists as separate and hers. The mother cannot exist without the baby, but this does not mean that the mother's identity is subsumed or erased.

This potentially adds a different interpretation to the attentiveness to the baby's body and needs discussed in previous chapters. While devotion to the baby's needs may reinforce dominant discourses of motherhood, it also potentially allows the mother to be present and to be remembered. Amara spent much time in interviews describing her stance of utter selflessness towards motherhood and her desire to be with her baby constantly. She would not even let other people hold her baby and described vigilantly watching so that she could fulfil her baby's every need. Her selflessness, however, is linked to her own maternal desires. After one description of conducting the daily tasks of motherhood with meticulous rhythm and painstaking attentiveness, she says:

And so my grandmother says that, *haai*, you mustn't do that; you must just leave her if she cries; she can cry there, right on the bed. And I say, 'mm-mm, as long as I am here, I am going to deal with her, because I am not working, I'm not doing, so I'll just spoil her' .... So that's why I said I don't mind, either I have to spoil her, I don't care, I will just spoil her. Mhm. Maybe I'll die next week, *ja*.

Amara's grandmother disapproves of her attentiveness, but Amara refuses to give it up. At this point, it is not primarily her baby's infection that she describes as motivating her attentiveness. What she is thinking of is her own infection and her transience as a mother: 'as long as I am here, I am going to deal with her.' It is her own position as a mother that is in jeopardy; being an HIV-positive mother in this moment means being as much of a mother as possible before one is a mother no longer. Her attentiveness allows her to make the most of the joys of motherhood before she has to give them up: 'maybe I'll die next week.' In the face of the loss of motherhood, the mother is both the child's mother and the mother of the child – both object and subject.

The mother is also potentially both mother and child – both the mother losing a child and the child losing the mother. This can be interpreted, for example, in Ayanda's accidental slip of the tongue when she identifies with her children contemplating her death. She says, 'it will be sad for me – for them'. Her self-correction resonates with her own sadness about having lost her mother, with her sadness about losing her children and with the sadness 'for me' of no longer being a living mother. Anele (whose mother is alive, but abandoned her as a child) describes a dream where she identifies with the pain of those left behind when a mother dies. This illustrates the interchangeability of mother and child:

Sometimes I dream. [pause] I don't dream of myself, you know. I dream of someone else that I love, you know, dying, and I can feel the pain, you know. Because last, last I dreamed of my mother; she was dead and I was very hurt, you know. I was very hurt; I was so hurt and I was scared and I woke up in the middle of the night; I was so scared, you know. I don't know why I was so scared, but maybe it was, it was not direct, you know, direct dream, but hey, I was very scared. So when I woke, I just thought about my kid, my child, that that's the feeling she is going to have when I die, you know.

Anele thinks that this was not a 'direct dream' – it was not only about the pain of losing her mother, but also about her child's pain. Her own pain in this dream is vivid and evokes the pain of identification between mother and child. She simultaneously feels her pain in losing a mother and her child's loss of her. Leleti contemplates not only the pain of her death for her child, but also for her mother. She is worried that her death will hurt her mother. She momentarily switches subject position to herself: 'sometimes I even feel that, no, sometimes I was not supposed to, to be dead and all that; I'll miss my mother.' Leleti is concerned about her mother and child missing her, but she is also concerned about how she will miss her mother when she is dead. Leleti and Anele access their own positions within motherhood through their mothers and children. The mother is the object of loss for her mother and child and is also the subject of loss of them and of herself.

CONCLUSION

From the mother's perspective, tragedy and joy are induced not only for the baby or the mother because of her baby, but also because she is a mother. This implies not only that the mother as subject exists, but also that it cannot be entirely separated from the maternal position of baby as subject. When dominant discourses of motherhood, and particularly of HIV-positive motherhood, require a silencing of the mother's voice, this does not require silencing a separate experience or position, but that women speaking within this discourse are required to erase an aspect of one interwoven position. If mother and baby are two sides of the same coin, speaking for the baby without speaking for the mother (for herself) does not imply a compartmentalisation of different subject positions, but requires a more active and violent process of trying to remove self from an interconnected equation of mother and baby.

Policy, research and practice seem to participate in these splits in two ways, firstly, by ignoring the mother through regarding the baby as central, and, secondly, by assuming these splits between mother and baby. A different perspective is required in which there is a recognition of both mother and baby that also allows for their interrelatedness. Mother and baby need to be recipients of treatment, for the sake of both. Integration of the treatment of mother and baby, in which mothers are considered as important as their babies, would offer more space for both mothers and babies. A broader acknowledgement of the contradictions of motherhood and the powerful emotions at play would be psychologically useful. Motherhood is important to the baby and the mother, and HIV-positive motherhood evokes both loss and joy. The experience of HIV-positive motherhood is tragic and painful, but it is also joyful and redemptive.

This returns one to the observation that it was easier for women to talk about themselves as HIV-positive than it was for them to talk about themselves as mothers. Similarly, it was easier for them to talk about motherhood in relation to, and from the perspective of, their babies than it was to talk about motherhood from their own perspective and position. This is in many ways precisely the position offered both in the broader literature about motherhood and in the popular imagination: a mother is known from the position of the child and is less knowable from the position of her subjectivity. Of course, Winnicott's formulation that 'there is no such thing as a baby' can be reversed to 'there is no such thing as a mother'. The baby is the thing that makes a mother a mother. There may, however, be meanings to 'there is no such thing as a mother' that do not only refer to the mother's connectedness to her baby. Such meanings may also refer to her alienation from being able to fully occupy the subject position of mother without slipping into seeing herself from the perspective of the other (not the (m)other, but the baby other).

For the HIV-positive mother, this becomes doubly determined by being in the socially constructed position of the damaged and damaging mother. The statement that 'there is no such thing as an HIV-positive mother' is simultaneously a statement about the mother's unimportance in light of the baby's well-being and a statement about the mother's absence. For each of these women, the knowledge that they would die – that they would become absent – was interconnected with the knowledge that their babies would have to suffer the loss of a mother. The fear that they may have infected their babies was a fear that they would have to suffer the loss of their babies, but also a fear that their babies would have to suffer a loss of self. The corresponding, irrational, fear that their babies may have infected them may represent a projected retaliation against themselves as mothers. To fully occupy the subject position of mother means to look at the baby and see the mother losing the baby as much as seeing the baby losing the mother.

9. Contradicting Maternity

HIV-positive motherhood is located within a collision of opposites. Folded into the same person are profound contradictions of creativity and destruction, hope and despair, good and bad, self and baby. For new mothers, the obligation and enjoyment of maternal care occupies the present, but awareness of the future is never far away, with all its uncertainties, except the knowledge of abandonment of some kind. This is complicated by social images of HIV-positive motherhood. Motherhood is contradictory in its own right, bringing expectations of virtue and purity of experience, but evoking the opposites of idealisation and denigration, power and powerlessness, creativity and destructiveness, with 'good' motherhood always on the brink of failure. HIV-positive identities are contradictory in a different way. The fantasised HIV-positive person is feared, evoking devastation and depravity. It seems that combining HIV-positive motherhood is incomprehensible and sets the mother apart from all other HIV-positive bodies. The contradictions of motherhood become solidified around the potential of the mother to damage her child and become hyperbolised in the popular and scientific imagination around death, guilt and abnormality. The HIV-positive mother amplifies social fantasies of both HIV and motherhood, but to become HIV-positive means grappling with the difference between this caricature and one's experience of oneself: it summons up gaps between social expectation and experience.

Recalling the photographs and scientific studies of HIV-positive motherhood presented in this book, the force with which fantasies of HIV-positive motherhood circulate in the social world becomes apparent. One way of reading *Contradicting Maternity* is through a comparison between these iconic social images of HIV-positive motherhood and the preoccupations of real HIV-positive mothers presented in chapters 5 to 8. This comparison foregrounds the fear resident in social images of HIV-positive motherhood and the associations of abjection they invoke. It is not just that HIV-positive motherhood is portrayed in relation to pathos: judgement and horror adhere to the fantasy such that the social fantasy returns the HIV-positive mother to a caricature who cannot be fully contemplated.

The fear of what the HIV-positive mother represents, of course, does not stand only in juxtaposition to the experiences of HIV-positive mothers recounted in this book. This fear was very much a part of the women's experiences and imagination about themselves and other HIV-positive mothers. In trying to make sense of themselves, there was a keen awareness of themselves as a representation of HIV-positive motherhood, as that abject thing that signifies danger. There was also, however, an array of other experiences and a range of possibilities for self: the representation resonated, but did not encapsulate.

In this sense, the HIV-positive mother is an object of fantasy and recipient of projections that divide the world into starkly split moral categories. This book has suggested, however, that taking up identities of motherhood and making sense of self both repeat and resist these contradictions. On the level of experience, mothers feared that they were guilty, blameworthy and damaging, not only in response to social fantasies, but also in response to personal fantasies elicited by the powerful fears and desires that HIV-positive motherhood evokes. Yet experience did not simply repeat social expectations. The contradictions experienced on the level of subjectivity were often between these expectations and the diversity of experience rather than within split social fantasies. There is a difference between social imagination and actual mothers: women did not simply repeat splits, but actively grappled with both good and bad.

The interlacing of personal and social meanings of HIV-positive motherhood, as well as the awareness of difference between self and other, inside and outside, have been central in understanding experiences of HIV-positive motherhood. The splits found in the public imagination – between personal and social and between self and other – were not characteristic of interview material. Rather, the women moved between personal and social, with one resonating against another, and comprehended themselves from the perspective of self as well as other. The method employed in listening to interview material was to specifically examine the movement between personal and social, self and other, in order to explore the experience of HIV-positive motherhood – i.e. the potential space between inner and outer reality (Winnicott, 1971). This focus on movement offsets the overwhelming tendency in existing research on HIV-positive motherhood to attempt to define stasis by looking for categories and definitions that exhaustively demarcate the HIV-positive mother. In practice, this meant listening to interview material for both discursive and psychodynamic meanings: for patterns of meaning linked to broader social discourses (which construct subjects and objects in a particular way within a system of power relations) and for anxieties, fears, fantasies and conflicts (which offer clues to particular psychodynamic meanings and processes).

Within interrelationships between personal and social meanings of HIV-positive motherhood, women constructed themselves, their babies and others in relation to discourses of motherhood and HIV. Many of the quotations presented can be read in terms of the productive circulation of power in ascribing self and body through discourse (Foucault, 1975). Interview data was replete with examples of the women looking at themselves, their babies or others through a social lens of meaning. At the same time, it has been suggested, the women were not simply spoken by discourse, but also entered into fantasies of themselves that were characterised by conflict, anxiety and defence. The realm of HIV-positive motherhood evokes powerful social meanings, but also powerful psychodynamic reverberations. Emotions were not simply inscribed by discourse, but were experienced in inner reality through the range of desire, fear, hatred, disgust, longing, joy, hope and love. Yet the focus of analysis was not on individual women and did not suggest complete uniqueness in response. These fantasies, conflicts, anxieties and emotions were unique to each woman, but also played out in a discursive realm that always drew back to how an HIV-positive mother *should* respond. It is this interrelationship between personal and social, of the mutual interactions between psychodynamic and discursive meaning, that seems particularly important in any attempt to understand the experience of HIV-positive motherhood. Acknowledging the discursive power through which HIV-positive mothers invest in particular discursive locations must be done in relation to an acknowledgement of the unconscious fantasies and affective responses that HIV-positive motherhood, in its extremes, elicits. Attention to only the former misses the inner reality of experience; attention to only the latter ignores the ways in which this inner experience is constituted by current discourses of HIV-positive motherhood. Between inner and outer reality lies a potential space where fluidity and play are possible (Winnicott, 1971). It is within this understanding that the analysis presented becomes an exploration of the terrain rather than a definition of HIV-positive motherhood.

Perhaps the constants in this terrain are the two central characters of mother and child. Another alternative way in which this book can be read is through the relationship between mother and child and the different perspectives that this dyad makes possible. It has been suggested that motherhood in general is dominated by the forepresence of the child and the relative absence of the mother: that mothers are expected to be absent from their own perspective and secondary to the needs of their babies. HIV-positive motherhood adds a particular dimension to this tendency to ignore the mother's subjectivity, because of the associations of damage that go with HIV-positive motherhood. This is illustrated in the dominant question in the popular and scientific imagination that concerns the well-being of the baby rather than the mother.

If HIV-positive motherhood is located within a collision of opposites, this is centrally played out in relation to the opposites of mother and baby. Mothers in this study felt these opposites. When talking about their babies, focus was often all-exclusive, with their own preoccupations put aside. Concern for their babies, particularly regarding their health and well-being, was clearly dominant. The baby's body was prioritised above the mother's body; care of and observation of baby overshadowed self. Yet maternal subjectivity was not absent and the importance to motherhood of the mother herself – of her desires, losses, hopes and fears – was experienced and lived. This aspect of HIV-positive motherhood is crucial to include precisely because it is so often missed.

Mother and baby, however, are indeed opposites of one another, but are also the opposite of that. While mother and baby were considered to have different needs and subjectivities, they were also at times interchangeable with each other. The status of the baby's body was often felt to determine the mother's body and the baby's well-being to determine the mother's. This was felt in reverse too – that the mother's body and mind predicted the baby's body and mind. This may be partly attributable to the possibility of a shared fate between mother and baby, underscored by the presence of HIV, but is also perhaps an insufficiently recognised dynamic of mother and baby as both subject and object. This interrelationship between mother and baby requires us to acknowledge both the difference and sameness of mother and baby at the level of experience. The mother looking at the baby looks at both herself and her other.

In considering the contradictions of HIV-positive maternity and in contradicting coexistent dominant discourses, these opposites of social fantasy versus experience, personal versus social and mother versus baby are informative. They are located, too, in the opposites evoked by the experience of HIV-positive motherhood – e.g. of life and death, tragedy and joy, hope and despair, good and bad. These opposites cannot entirely be reconciled, but neither can one side of an opposition entirely negate the other. Broader tropes of motherhood are repeated, dodged or evaded in interviews, but they do not entirely separate from their reverse and neither do they encapsulate the experience of motherhood.

This book has presented an analysis of the multiplicity of motherhood through an analysis of experience emerging through the different bodies and voices of the HIV-positive mother. Through this analysis, it has become clear that dominant discourses of motherhood recursively call upon the subject to be selfless, faceless and silent in service of the baby, but that a position of resistance exists in which the mothers' desires and fears are central. Perhaps because of the centrality of infection and death to constructions of HIV-positive motherhood, and perhaps also because of the brutality with which discourse separates person from mother and mother from baby, these desires and fears are played out on the body and in stories only in enclaves and often through splits and opposites. 'Contradicting maternity' operates as a metaphor that evokes the discursive imperative to erase this position, while at the same time both celebrating and mourning both baby and mother.

An almost insurmountable gap for the women in this study seemed to be between HIV personhood and motherhood. Spoken about separately, kept separate from one another, being HIV-positive was differentiated from being an HIV-positive mother. The first concerns one's own infection and its implications for oneself; the second is located in the relationship between mother and baby. The women positioned themselves differently in relation to different aspects of identity, and each of these positions held somewhat different implications for subjectivity. The split between HIV-positive *person* (as gendered or as HIV infected) and HIV-positive *mother* (as secondary to the baby or as a mother in her own right) suggests a repetition of the incomprehensibility of HIV-positive motherhood. One's own infection is irreconcilable with identities of motherhood and possible infection of one's baby.

However, this gap between person and mother was not a repetition of constructions of motherhood in which the baby is primary and the mother invisible. It is not the case that women were subjects as HIV-positive *person* and objects as HIV-positive *mother*. On the contrary, the women were both subject and object. As *HIV-positive*, the women simultaneously spoke as HIV-positive subjects and were positioned as objects within discourses and in relation to others. Contrary to social expectations, the *mothers* were not entirely turned away from themselves towards their babies, although their babies held a special place and were considered to be more important than themselves. From the perspective of motherhood, both mother and baby were both subject and object.

It could be suggested that the gap between person and mother, rather than implying differential positions as HIV-positive subject and maternal object, strives to keep contamination of subjectivity in abeyance. Being constructed as an object (HIV-positive or maternal) informs one's subjectivity, but taking up the position of speaking subject requires identification and, sometimes, defensive protection. To speak as an HIV-positive person risks one's maternal position both as object to one's baby and maternal subject: the irreconcilability is that each position requires a different kind of subject, one as infected and the other as maternal and infecting. Similarly, to speak from the maternal position means to acknowledge the insertion of HIV into the mother–infant relationship and into the experience of motherhood. There is enough to contemplate without the addition of one's own HIV-positive body or the partnership that created both HIV and the baby. Keeping them separate limits infection.

In contrast to the consideration of one's own HIV-positive infection, motherhood involves primary thought about the baby. This is characterised by uncertainty and breathlessness, with discourse failing to help in the incessant search for infection on the baby's body. HIV insinuates itself into the mother–infant relationship and becomes an almost physical presence between mother and baby – 'almost', because it operates in the unknown and evokes a tragedy that goes beyond comprehensibility. The normal anxieties and fantasies of motherhood become channelled and interpreted through HIV. The potentiality of the virus leaves space for little else and therefore prompts a desperate desire for everything else to be good. Looking at their babies, fantasies of HIV-positive motherhood in the social world vie for position against the desire of the women to be good mothers to their babies. In this way, maternal subjectivity vacillates between the splits enacted in broader discourses of motherhood – between the good and bad mother, the damaging and caring mother, the close and distant mother – while maternal practice strives towards the attainment of the ideal.

THE MOTHER OF A BABY: A SECONDARY POSITION

In this process, the baby's body occupies centre stage and the potentiality of infection, despite the odds being stacked in the baby's favour, absorbs the mother's mind. This is often in the context of uncertainty and the lack of knowledge regarding whether or not the baby is HIV infected. The mothers described careful scrutiny of their baby's bodies, searching for signs of HIV and simultaneously for signs of health. Trying to read their babies through their knowledge of themselves and through their observation of their babies bodies is inevitably a process of fantasy through which anything can transform into its reverse. Any observation (of a rash, a swollen gland, a good appetite) can signify either tragedy or joy, death or life. Despite constant imagination about what the baby's body might mean, women often expressed a constriction of imagination regarding their babies, e.g. only expressing fantasies of illness after a point of safety had been reached. This suggests a dual process of constantly imagining and strictly limiting imagination to thinking only what is manageable. In this process, medicine offered solace and reassurance, but often left an excess that could not quite be contained, precisely because medical intervention could not bridge the gap between mother and baby. When the women were finally able to state with certainty whether or not their babies were HIV infected, the relief from this state of uncertainty was enormous and a different space could be entertained between mother and baby that was not dominated by HIV. The hard-won state of certainty when the women knew the fates of their babies was articulated with awe and cherished as a salvation for both themselves and their babies. Even then, however, the possibility of HIV infection was rejected with difficulty and continued to return. The possibility of reversals remained.

This underscores the extent to which the mothers were concerned about their babies and the extent to which early motherhood was characterised by preoccupation with the well-being of their babies. All the mothers expressed this concern and preoccupation and all grappled with the tenuousness of trying to make sense of whether their babies were safe or in danger. The concentration with which the mother's mind was focused on minding the baby's body indicates the extent to which the baby is prioritised, as well as the acuteness of the mother's awareness of what she may have done to her baby. Clear links can be made to dominant discourses regarding the all-primacy of the baby in the mother–infant relationship, as well as regarding the urgency involved and the danger of HIV-positive motherhood to babies. In minding the baby's body, the presence of these particular configurations of power are inescapable. There was also a quality to maternal reflections on the baby's body, however, that was beyond words and not simply inscribed by discourse. The love that the mothers expressed towards their babies, their desire to protect them from HIV – and consequently from themselves – and their anxiety regarding the fate of their babies contributed to a sense of breathlessness and unarticulability in their reflections. This is no doubt exploded by dominant discourses regarding HIV-positive motherhood. What plays out on the baby's body is a microcosm of the drama of self and other, inside and outside, salvation and condemnation, where the fantasies and anxieties of HIV-positive motherhood interact with social discourses that inscribe the baby's body.

The mother–infant relationship serves as another site where HIV and anxieties about HIV-positive motherhood dominate. This relationship is characterised by the everyday tasks of caring for a baby: in feeding and holding, watching the baby learn to crawl, attending to the baby's delight and distress. This aspect of early motherhood has its own language, which is often sensuous and non-verbal. The fear of HIV added its own language to the early mother–infant relationship for HIV-positive mothers. The women described a heightening of maternal attentiveness, as if watchfulness could ward off the possibility of infection and the anxiety of being an HIV-positive mother. Chapter 6 offered two extreme examples of maternal protectiveness. Lukanyo felt her overweight baby to be a barometer of good maternal care, her feeding of her infant a way of defending against the anxiety that she may have infected him. Dikeledi's fear of infection outlasted her baby's HIV-negative test result, the intensity of which was communicated to him so that he would not even put a cheese curl in his mouth without her approval. These extreme examples illustrate the power of maternal attentiveness, its felt importance and possible explanations regarding what it protects against. There were many less extreme examples in interview discussions, where women spoke about their alertness to their interactions with their babies and their feelings that they needed to be particularly good mothers to make up for the possibility of infection of their baby or of their own deaths.

In moments of thought about their babies, too, HIV intervened and made its presence felt. Thinking about their child's character, smile or attempts to crawl, for example, turned from pride or consideration into concern about HIV in an instant. HIV held pride of place between mother and infant, such that the everyday interactions between mother and baby could be interrupted, particularly by anxieties regarding the baby's health or future. Maternal guilt was also channelled specifically in relation to HIV: Boitumelo's forgotten bottle signified not only bad motherhood to her, but also a maternal slip that could result in the intervention of HIV. Her feeling of guilt was overlaid both with social images of the maternal ideal and of HIV-positive maternal threat. In this way, HIV mediated motherhood, adding its colour to minute interactions.

Breastfeeding represented a particular dilemma for the mothers, given its potentially infecting associations with HIV. The quiet insistence with which the women expressed their refusal to breastfeed indicates the extent to which medical advice was taken on board. Given how difficult it is not to breastfeed in this particular cultural landscape, the insistence on refraining from breastfeeding resonates too with the urgency the women felt in practising good motherhood. This was not an uncomplicated decision for many of the women, who felt the loss of breastfeeding both for themselves and their babies. As a potent absence signalling the presence of HIV, the women felt deprived of this experience of motherhood both for themselves (the primary position of motherhood) and for their babies (the secondary position of motherhood). Foreshadowed, however, was a fear of doing the wrong thing, and this was sometimes felt in relation to both the act of breastfeeding and the decision not to breastfeed. Women were concerned that breastfeeding would lead to the loss of their babies, but refraining from breastfeeding represented a variety of losses as well. Overtly, women were concerned about the losses that this decision would bring to their baby's health, as well as to the quality of their attachment relationships. This presents one example of many concerning the layers of loss that HIV-positive motherhood offers and the impossibility of avoiding feelings of guilt. Either direction leads to questions; answers cannot be pinned down. Fantasies of the baby and of the mother–infant relationship are characterised by tensions and losses that require repeated checking and repeated thought.

GOOD OR BAD MOTHER?

A primary tension between mother and baby concerned the question of whether the women were good mothers or bad mothers. It is clear that the mothers acutely felt themselves to be both – at different times and at the same time. The concern to practice maternity with care and conscientiousness pervaded interviews as intensely as the fear of failed motherhood. These opposites preoccupied the mothers, but all were uneasily settled. A moment could turn a feeling into its opposite. The mothers were keenly aware of themselves as mothers and diligently self-monitoring. It is important to understand this process in terms of the currents of experience of HIV-positive motherhood and not as evidence of their actual parenting. Feeling like a good or bad mother is not the same as objectively being good or bad. It might be possible to conclude from interviews that the women were sensitively aware; one may equally construct an argument that they were hypersensitive, overprotective and insecure in their mothering. It is certainly the case that maternal awareness was keenly expressed and that the women felt their maternal adequacy to be important. The care with which they considered the bodies and development of their babies, as well as their interactions with their babies, indicates the extent to which they were sensitive to maternal practice.

Yet, although the focus of this book is not on whether HIV-positive mothers are good or bad mothers, it was evident that some were good and some were bad. This diversity indicates the absurdity of asking whether or not HIV-positive mothers are good or bad: a type or category of HIV-positive motherhood does not exist. HIV status may certainly influence motherhood, in interaction with different issues for different women, but it is not all-defining or characteristic.

The women often brought their babies to interviews, bringing live mother–infant interaction into the room. The opportunity to observe these minute interactions indicated that many of the mothers were attuned to their babies' needs and responsive in their care. The rhythm when the baby cried or laughed was assumed and interacted. Some of the women were better at this than others. Two of the women, in particular, were clearly clinically depressed, and this could be observed in mother–infant interaction. For the first woman, who verbalised thoughts about killing both herself and her baby, her baby's cries during one interview could not be quelled and she was consistently unresponsive to her baby's state. The second woman, who was severely depressed, stared blankly at her baby's equally blank face, and it seemed apparent that her baby had given up responding to an unresponsive mother. The depression of both of these women, no doubt, was heavily influenced by their HIV diagnosis. It would be a mistake, however, to say that they were unresponsive mothers because they were depressed because they were HIV-positive. There were clearly a number of other factors at play. This is an obvious statement: HIV-positive mothers cannot be bad mothers simply because they are HIV-positive. Yet this is often what research implies when it frames questions about (bad) HIV-positive motherhood. With all their variations, however, all the mothers (even the two very depressed ones) spoke spontaneously and with conviction about their desire to be good mothers. Although it is not possible (and should not be possible) to conclude from this book that HIV-positive mothers evidence particular kinds of parenting, it is clear that the mothers interviewed here are not negligent mothers who foster bad attachments because of their lack of interest in motherhood or their lack of motivation to mother their children. Acutely aware of the presence of HIV in the mother–infant relationship, the women also strove to curb the threat of HIV to the mother–infant relationship, and to their babies in particular.

THE MOTHER HERSELF: A PRIMARY POSITION

Where the primary preoccupation was in taking the baby's needs as of greatest consequence, interviews included the more hidden identity of the mother from the mother's perspective. The mother is not only an object to her baby, but a subject in her own right, with her own maternal desires and fears and her own subjectivity. This position was largely on the edges of interview material, but the powerful fears and desires of the mother-herself makes this position far from marginal, and certainly not absent. Kaplan (1992: 3) describes the mother's position as an 'absent presence'; for the women in this study it was more like a present absence. The maternal body, for example, was far from central, but the ways in which it emerged in interviews suggest its inscription by and resistance of social constructions of motherhood. Further, each mother was not selflessly turned away from herself, but engaged with her love of her baby as well as with her anger and fear related to the baby and with the loss of herself both to her baby and for herself.

The maternal body, as that which is distinctly the mother's own, offered a site upon which the ambiguities of maternal subjectivity were enacted. Although the maternal body was only present in moments of interviews, its power asserted itself as a body upon which discursive imperatives were deployed and also as one that resisted these imperatives in its expression of maternal meaning. This doubling of the maternal body – as a place to police maternity and as an expression of the joyful and forbidden aspects of maternity for the mother herself – offers a microcosm of HIV-positive motherhood and its tensions between social and personal meanings of self. In this sense, the maternal body is a fraught location, but one that offers a container for maternity in between inner and outer reality and in between mother and baby.

The four sites where the maternal body found expression were to be found on the margins of interview material, but their marginality was replete with meaning. The maternal body was almost visible in its absence, expressing itself in the subtext of conversation, as in Bongiwe's contemplation of her baby's infectedness and infectiousness. In considering her baby, her partner and herself, it is her maternal body, as potentially infecting and also as potentially procreative, that expresses the possibilities and anxieties of her own position of motherhood. The connections among the maternal body, the HIV-positive body and the baby's body also become visible, for it is at the moment that the woman's body also becomes a maternal body that the threat of HIV for both mother and baby can be seen.

Secondly, the maternal body was visible in moments when maternal infectiousness was most gruesome: in the moment of birth or when blood bridged the boundary between mother and baby in mother–infant interaction. It is particularly striking that these images hardly featured in interview material, given the power of the descriptions of other things that were to be found. The ability of the imagination to rob the speaker of words in the face of the maternal body giving birth, for example, underscores the possible associations between the maternal body and the terror of infection.

In contrast to the almost unmentioned maternal body in relation to self, the maternal body was most visible through the stories the women told about other women. Here, there were clear splits in how the women imagined other HIV-positive maternal bodies: either in relation to good, idyllic mothers (like those seen at the hospital) or in relation to bad, dangerous mothers who were HIV-positive, but continued to breastfeed or procreate. Behind the image of the good, idyllic HIV-positive mother was a series of injunctions to the self: in order to be good too, one had to be like these other good mothers and to strictly adhere to the selflessness they represented. Comparisons took place in relation to what one should not do. For example, one should not give one's baby up for adoption and one should not allow room for the possibility of abortion. In these 'shoulds', glimpses could be found of both the innocence of babies and their potential dangerousness, as well as the guilt of mothers who wanted things for themselves. The images of bad HIV-positive mothers, who breastfeed or procreate, potentially allowed the women some expression of their guilt and fears, but in projected forms. The horror and disgust with which the women routinely spoke about others breastfeeding or procreating are commensurate with the fear evoked by the HIV-positive maternal body (symbolised in the posture of breastfeeding) and its links to sexuality (symbolised by the procreative body) and to fantasies of deliberate destructiveness through causing the baby's death by breastfeeding or procreating. It seems significant that bad mothers were limited in their portrayal to these two actions, indicating the extremes of what the maternal body is capable of enacting.

The fourth place where the maternal body was evoked was through the baby, and particularly through the vexed question of whether or not the baby had been infected by the mother. This seems like an obvious connection to make, and concerns regarding the possibility of the mother infecting the baby were pervasive. However, the more direct connection between the maternal body and infectiousness was also one that occupied the margins of interviews. The form that this concern took indicates the extent of relatedness between mother and baby: in the form of the power of the baby's body to symbolically change the body of the mother. If the baby was safe from HIV, the mother could feel safe too. Conversely, if the baby was at risk, maternal risk was correspondingly amplified. It was not only guilt that forged these relationships, but also experience, through maternal awareness of the interconnected fate of mother and baby. The division between mother and baby so often found in conceptions of HIV-positive motherhood and babyhood, then, belies the experience of motherhood from the mother's perspective, in which mother and baby are interchangeable and where creativity and destructiveness are bi-directional in the mother–infant relationship.

Where the mother's body indicated the occupation of primary maternal subjectivity – maternity from the experience of the mother – the mothers' voices also spoke about this experience. '*Thula mama*' operates as a metaphor not only for the silencing of the maternal voice, but also for its expression: its consolation of pain and its expression of joy. Although the mothers spoke with difficulty about themselves as mothers, turning away from themselves towards the centrality of their babies, they also spoke about their own maternal experiences: their fears and desires for themselves. Within the shadow of HIV, the maternal voice was bound to its implications for their own experience of mothering, but was also defiant against the threat HIV represents.

The intervention of HIV means that some aspects of maternity are more easily expressed than others. The more difficult aspects of maternal experience – anger and hate in particular – could be mentioned, but seldom dwelled upon. The threat of one's own anger or hatred dovetails with the threat of HIV. The existence of legitimate anger and expected fantasies of destroying or being destroyed by one's baby interlaces with the destructiveness represented by HIV. This is an aspect of motherhood that belongs to the mother. As Roszika Parker (1995: 20–21) comments:

> Now, of course, there are many reasons why guilt works to split love and hate so far apart that love ceases to mitigate hate, but a primary cause is our culture's ambivalence towards maternal ambivalence .... For parents and non-parents alike, ambivalence about ambivalence is based on the terror that hate will always destroy love and lead to isolation and abandonment. Our culture defends itself against the recognition of ambivalence originating in the mother by denigrating or idealising her. A denigrated mother is simply hateful and has no love for the child to lose. An idealised mother is hate-free, constant and unreal.

Threatening in the general domain of motherhood, partly because discourses of motherhood require an all-good mother, it seems that discourses of HIV explode this danger. There is an aspect of being an HIV-positive mother that elicits internal fears about the danger of anything but love. Discourses of HIV-positive motherhood, however, collude with this fear and turn it into a kind of reality. Voicing one's own maternity is limited by understandings of HIV-positive motherhood as dangerous and deadly. Different representations may not solve internal fears of destructiveness, but would undoubtedly open the potential space between mother and child so that these feelings could be legitimated.

The link between HIV-positive motherhood and destructiveness, then, belongs both in the expected fantasies of individual women and in the meanings generated in the social world. Its associations to life and death exist in potentiality, since actual death is as yet unknown and cannot be judged. This is helped by medication in reality, where the possibility exists that life can be considerably extended. Maternity, however, is crucially about making life and then nurturing its fragility. From the perspective of the mother, it is also about being alive oneself to enjoy the experience of motherhood. These divisions between life and death are complicated by divisions between mother and baby. In Nonyameko's striking story, where she believed herself to be cured of HIV because her baby was HIV-negative, and therefore able to procreate again, the implications of life and death in the context of HIV can be seen to play themselves out not in the division between mother and baby, but in the interchangeability of mother and baby. The possibility of salvation is both for herself and for her baby, and allows her to imagine having another baby. Fantasies of life and death play out in the connectedness between mother and baby and not just in the mother's individual and private subjectivity.

The mothers' desires and fears are narrated not only through desires and fears for their babies, but also through the interchangeability of mother and baby and the interconnectedness of motherhood with HIV infection and death. Death, which has pervaded the analysis, disrupts the oppositions and leaves a surplus to be explained. Its own opposite – life or love or joy – operates similarly and is also not its opposite. And thus the analysis presented, based as it is on words and stories, exists uneasily between the tragedy of motherhood from the mother's perspective and maternal pride, defiance and joy. Analysis suggested an interchangeability between mother and baby such that each could be both infected and infecting, saved and damned. The fluidity of maternity suggests that divisions between mother-of-baby and mother-herself, while enacted, are artificial. The mother is turned away from herself and her baby; turned towards herself and her baby; and the baby is both the central subject in the mother–infant dyad and an object within the mother's own fantasies. Two mothers exist, therefore, and two babies; two tragedies and two joys; and then the violence of social splits between them, as well as the violence of HIV.

Appendix:
Interview Content

Interviews aimed to cover the following areas of experience:

The experience of receiving an HIV-positive diagnosis
The implications of being diagnosed while pregnant
Disclosure: who had been told and why/not; experiences of disclosure
How women believed that they had become HIV-positive and the meanings that these explanations had for them
Relationship to the father of the baby and the father's experience of parenthood
Conceptions of the future for themselves and their children
What motherhood meant to them
If this was their first child, what this meant to them. If a second or subsequent child, how they thought motherhood was similar to and/or different from their previous experiences
How they evaluated themselves as mothers
Hopes and fears about motherhood
Discussion about the pregnancy and/or the baby
Thoughts on breastfeeding
Implications of the delay in knowing the baby's status
Thoughts and feelings about the baby's status
Emotions, fantasies and dreams about HIV and motherhood
Experiences of coming to the clinic and seeing other HIV-positive mothers
Experiences of the perceptions of others (including other mothers and HIV-positive and -negative people)
Family background
Experience of the interview

Biographical and demographic information (age; employment status; living circumstances; time of diagnosis; partner status; number of other children; baby's status, if known) was elicited during the course of interviews at points appropriate to the discussion.

Bibliography

Antle, B., L. Wells, R. Goldie, D. DeMatteo & S. King. 2001. 'Challenges of parenting for families living with HIV/AIDS.' *Social Work*, 46(2): 159–69.

Armistead, L., E. Morse, R. Forehand, P. Morse & L. Clark. 1999. 'African-American women and self-disclosure of HIV infection: Rates, predictors, and relationship to depressive symptomatology.' *AIDS and Behavior*, 3(3): 195–204.

Armistead, L., L. Tannenbaum, R. Forehand, E. Morse & P. Morse. 2001. 'Disclosing HIV status: Are mothers telling their children?' *Journal of Pediatric Psychology*, 26(1): 11–20.

Badinter, E. 1981. *The Myth of Motherhood: An Historical View of the Maternal Instinct.* London: Souvenir Press.

Barrett, G. & C. R. Victor. 1994. '"We just want to be a normal family ...": Paediatric HIV/AIDS services at an inner-London teaching hospital.' *AIDS Care*, 6(4): 423–33.

Barthes, R. 1980; republished 2000. *Camera Lucida: Reflections on Photography.* London: Vintage.

Benedek, T. 1959. 'Parenthood as a developmental phase: A contribution to libido theory.' *Journal of the American Psychoanalytic Association*, 7: 389–417.

Benjamin, W. 1935. 'The work of art in the age of mechanical reproduction.' Repr. in G. Mast, M. Cohen & L. Braudy (eds). 1992. *Film Theory and Criticism*, 4th ed. New York & Oxford: Oxford University Press.

Bennetts, A., N. Shaffer, C. Manopaiboon, P. Chaiyakul, W. Siriwasin, P. Mock, K. Klumthanom, S. Sorapipatana, C. Yuvasevee, S. Jalanchavanapate & L. Clark. 1999. 'Determinants of depression and HIV-related worry among HIV-positive women who have recently given birth, Bangkok, Thailand.' *Social Science and Medicine*, 49: 737–49.

Berger, J. 1972. *Ways of Seeing*. London: British Broadcasting Corporation & Penguin Books.

Berryman, J. 1991. 'Perspectives on later motherhood.' In A. Phoenix, A. Woollett & E. Lloyd (eds). *Motherhood: Meanings, Practices and Ideologies*, pp. 103–22. London: Sage.

Bibring, G., T. Dwyer, D. Huntington & A. Valenstein. 1961a. 'A study of the psychological processes in pregnancy and of the earliest mother–child relationship, I: Some propositions and comments.' *The Psychoanalytic Study of the Child*, XVI: 9–24.

Bibring, G., T. Dwyer, D. Huntington & A. Valenstein. 1961b. 'A study of the psychological processes in pregnancy and of the earliest mother–child relationship, II: Methodological considerations.' *The Psychoanalytic Study of the Child*, XVI: 25–72.

Biggar, H. & R. Forehand. 1998. 'The relationship between maternal HIV status and child depressive symptoms: Do maternal depressive symptoms play a role?' *Behavior Therapy*, 29(3): 409–22.

Biggar, H., R. Forehand, M. W. Chance, E. Morse, P. Morse & M. Stock. 2000. 'The relationship of maternal HIV status and home variables to academic performance of African American children.' *Aids and Behavior*, 4(3): 241–52.

Billig, M. 1999. *Freudian Repression*. Cambridge: Cambridge University Press.

Birksted-Breen, D. 2000. 'The experience of having a baby: A developmental view.' In J. Raphael-Leff (ed.). *'Spilt Milk': Perinatal Loss and Breakdown*, pp. 17–27. London: Institute of Psychoanalysis.

Black, M., P. Nair & D. Harrington. 1994. 'Maternal HIV infection: Parenting and early child development.' *Journal of Pediatric Psychology*, 19(5): 595–616.

Bland, R. M., N. C. Rollins, A. Coutsoudis & H. M. Coovadia. 2002. 'Breastfeeding practices in an area of high HIV prevalence in rural South Africa.' *Acta Paediatrica*, 91(6): 704–11.

Bradley, E. 2000. 'Pregnancy and the internal world.' In J. Raphael-Leff (ed.). *'Spilt Milk': Perinatal Loss and Breakdown*, pp. 28–38. London: Institute of Psychoanalysis.

Breen, D. 1975. *The Birth of a First Child: Towards an Understanding of Femininity*. London: Tavistock.

Breen, D. 1989. *Talking with Mothers*. London: Free Association Books.

Brink, E. 1990. 'Man-made women: Gender, class and the ideology of the *volksmoeder*.' In C. Walker (ed.). *Women and Gender in Southern Africa to 1945*, pp. 273–92. Cape Town: David Philip.

Butler, J. 1990. *Gender Trouble: Feminism and the Subversion of Identity*. London & New York: Routledge.

Butler, J. 1993. *Bodies that Matter: On the Discursive Limits of 'Sex'.* London & New York: Routledge.

Butler, J. 1997. *The Psychic Life of Power: Theories of Subjection*. Stanford: Stanford University Press.

Caplan, P. J. 1990. 'Making mother-blaming visible: The emperor's new clothes.' In J. P. Knowles & E. Cole (eds). *Woman-defined Motherhood*, pp. 61–70. New York & London: Harrington Park Press.

Chalfin, S. R., C. L. Grus & L. Tomaszeski. 2002. 'Caregiver's stress secondary to raising young children with HIV infection: A preliminary investigation.' *Journal of Clinical Psychology in Medical Settings*, 9(3): 211–18.

Chesler, P. 1990. 'Mother-hatred and mother-blaming: What Electra did to Clytemnestra.' In J. P. Knowles & E. Cole (eds). *Woman-defined Motherhood*, pp. 71–82. New York & London: Harrington Park Press.

Chodorow, N. 1978. *The Reproduction of Mothering: Psychoanalysis and the Sociology of Gender*. California: University of California Press.

Christian, B. 1994. 'An angle of seeing: Motherhood in Buchi Emecheta's *Joys of Motherhood* and Alice Walker's *Meridian*.' In E. N. Glenn, G. Chang & L. R. Forcey (eds). *Mothering: Ideology, Experience, and Agency*, pp. 95–120. New York & London: Routledge.

Coutsoudis, A. 2005. 'Breastfeeding and the HIV positive mother: The debate continues.' *Early Human Development*, 81(1): 87–93.

Coutsoudis, A., K. Pillay, E. Spooner, H. M. Coovadia, L. Pembrey & M. Newell. 2003. 'Morbidity in children born to women infected with human immunodeficiency virus in South Africa: Does mode of feeding matter?' *Acta Paediatrica*, 92(8): 890–95.

Coward, R. 1997. 'The heaven and hell of mothering: Mothering and ambivalence in the mass media.' In W. Hollway & B. Featherstone (eds). *Mothering and Ambivalence*, pp. 111–18. London: Routledge.

Dally, A. 1982. *Inventing Motherhood: The Consequences of an Ideal*. London: Burnett Books.

Daniels, D. 2004. 'They need to know where they came from to appreciate where they are going to: Visual commentary of informal settlement women on motherhood.' *JENdA: A Journal of Culture and African Women Studies*, 5. <http://www.jendajournal. com/issue5/daniels.htm>.

D'Auria, J., B. Christian & M. Shandor Miles. 2006. 'Being there for my baby: Early responses of HIV-infected mothers with an HIV-exposed infant.' *Journal of Pediatric Health Care*, 20(1): 11–18.

Davies, B. 1990. 'The problem of desire.' *Social Problems*, 37(4): 501–16.

Davies, B. & R. Harré. 1990. 'Positioning: The discursive production of selves.' *Journal for the Theory of Social Behaviour*, 20(1): 43–63.

DeMarco, R., M. M. Lynch & R. Board. 2002. 'Mothers who silence themselves: A concept with clinical implications for women living with HIV/AIDS and their children.' *Journal of Pediatric Nursing*, 17(2): 89–95.

Department of Health. 2002. *Interim Findings on the National PMTCT Pilot Sites: Lessons and Recommendations*. <http://www.doh.co.za>.

Department of Health. 2006. *National HIV and Syphilis Antenatal Sero-prevalence Survey in South Africa 2005*. <http://www.doh.co.za>.

Deutsch, H. 1945. *The Psychology of Women*. New York: Grune & Stratton.

Dinnerstein, D. 1977. *The Mermaid and the Minotaur: Sexual Arrangements and Human Malaise*. New York: Harper Colophon Books.

Dorsey, S., R. Forehand, L. Armistead, E. Morse, P. Morse & M. Stock. 1999. 'Mother knows best? Mother and child report of behavioural difficulties of children of HIV-infected mothers.' *Journal of Psychopathology and Behavioral Assessment*, 21(3): 191–206.

Duncan, N. & B. Rock. 1997. 'Going beyond the statistics.' In B. Rock (ed.). *Spirals of Suffering*, pp. 69–113. Pretoria: Human Sciences Research Council.

Du Toit, M. 2003. 'The domesticity of Afrikaner nationalism: *Volksmoeders* and the ACVV, 1904–1929.' *Journal of Southern African Studies*, 29(1): 155–76.

Elliott, A. & S. Frosh. 1995. *Psychoanalysis in Contexts: Paths between Theory and Modern Culture*. London: Routledge.

Elliott, A. & C. Spezzano. 2000. *Psychoanalysis at Its Limits: Navigating the Postmodern Turn*. London & New York: Free Association Books.

Elliott, R., C. T. Fischer & D. L. Rennie. 1999. 'Evolving guidelines for publication of qualitative research studies in psychology and related fields.' *British Journal of Clinical Psychology*, 38: 215–29.

Emecheta, B. 1979. *The Joys of Motherhood*. Oxford: Heinemann.

Etchegoyen, A. 1997. 'Inhibition of mourning and the replacement child syndrome.' In J. Raphael-Leff & R. Perelberg (eds). *Female Experience: Three Generations of British Women Psychoanalysts on Work with Women*, pp. 195–218. London: Routledge.

Family Health Project Research Group. 1998. 'The Family Health Project: A multidisciplinary longitudinal investigation of children whose mothers are HIV-infected.' *Clinical Psychology Review*, 18(7): 839–56.

Featherstone, B. 1997. 'Introduction: Crisis in the Western family.' In W. Hollway & B. Featherstone (eds). *Mothering and Ambivalence*, pp. 1–16. London: Routledge.

Flax, J. 1993. *Disputed Subjects: Essays on Psychoanalysis, Politics and Philosophy*. New York & London: Routledge.

Forehand, R., R. Steele, L. Armistead, E. Morse, P. Simon & L. Clark. 1998. 'The Family Health Project: Psychosocial adjustment of children whose mothers are HIV infected.' *Journal of Consulting and Clinical Psychology*, 66(3): 513–20.

Forsyth, B., L. Damour, S. Nagler & J. Adnopoz. 1996. 'The psychological effects of parental human immunodeficiency virus infection on uninfected children.' *Archives of Pediatrics and Adolescent Medicine*, 150(10): 1015–20.

Foucault, M. 1971. 'The order of discourse.' In R. Young (ed.). *Untying the Text: A Post-Structuralist Reader*, pp. 48–78. Boston & London: Routledge.

Foucault, M. 1975. *Discipline and Punish: The Birth of the Prison*. London: Penguin.

Frizele, K. & G. Hayes. 1999. 'Experiences of motherhood: Challenging ideals.' *Psychology in Society*, 25: 17–36.

Frosh, S. 1997a. *For and against Psychoanalysis*. London: Routledge.

Frosh, S. 1997b. 'Fathers' ambivalence (too).' In W. Hollway & B. Featherstone (eds). *Mothering and Ambivalence*, pp. 37–53. London: Routledge.

Frosh, S. 2002. *After Words: The Personal in Gender, Culture and Psychotherapy*. London: Palgrave.

Frosh, S., A. Phoenix & R. Pattman. 2000. '"But it's racism I really hate": Young masculinities, racism and psychoanalysis.' *Psychoanalytic Psychology*, 17: 225–42.

Frosh, S., A. Phoenix & R. Pattman. 2003. 'Taking a stand: Using psychoanalysis to explore the positioning of subjects in discourse.' *British Journal of Social Psychology*, 42: 39–53.

Gallop, R. M., W. J. Lancee, G. Taerk, R. A. Coates & M. Fanning. 1992. 'Fear of contagion and AIDS: Nurses' perception of risk.' *AIDS Care: Psychological and Socio-Medical Aspects of AIDS/HIV*, 4(1): 103–9.

Gentzler, E. 1993. *Contemporary Translation Theories*. London & New York: Routledge.

Glenn, E. N. 1994. 'Social constructions of mothering: A thematic overview.' In E. N. Glenn, G. Chang & L. R. Forcey (eds). *Mothering: Ideology, Experience, and Agency*, pp. 1–32. New York & London: Routledge.

Greene, B. 1990. 'Sturdy bridges: The role of African-American mothers in the socialization of African-American children.' In J. P. Knowles & E. Cole (eds). *Woman-defined Motherhood*, pp. 205–26. New York & London: Harrington Park Press.

Guy, J. 1990. 'Gender oppression in Southern Africa's precapitalist societies.' In C. Walker (ed.). *Women and Gender in Southern Africa to 1945*, pp. 33–47. Cape Town: David Philip.

Hale, A. K., D. Holditch-Davis, J. D'Auria & M. S. Miles. 1999. 'The usefulness of an assessment of emotional involvement of HIV-positive mothers and their infants.' *Journal of Pediatric Health Care*, 13(5): 230–36.

Harrison, A. & E. Montgomery. 2001. 'Life histories, reproductive histories: Rural South African women's narratives of fertility, reproductive health and illness.' *Journal of Southern African Studies*, 27(2): 311–28.

Heath, J. & M. Rodway. 1999. 'Psychosocial needs of women infected with HIV.' *Social Work in Health Care*, 29(3): 43–57.

Henriques, J., W. Hollway, C. Urwin, C. Venn & V. Walkerdine (eds). 1984. *Changing the Subject: Psychology, Social Regulation and Subjectivity*. London & New York: Methuen.

Hogan, K. 1998. 'Gendered visibilities in black women's AIDS narratives.' In N. L. Roth & K. Hogan (eds). *Gendered Epidemic: Representations of Women in the Age of AIDS*, pp. 165–90. London: Routledge.

Hollway, W. 1989. *Subjectivity and Method in Psychology: Gender, Meaning and Science*. London: Sage.

Hollway, W. & T. Jefferson. 2000. *Doing Qualitative Research Differently: Free Association, Narrative and the Interview Method*. London: Sage.

Hoosen, S. & A. Collins. 2004. 'Sex, sexuality and sickness: Discourses of gender and HIV/AIDS among KwaZulu-Natal women.' *South African Journal of Psychology*, 34(3): 487–505.

Horney, K. 1967. *Feminine Psychology*. London: Routledge.

Hough, E. S., G. Brumitt, T. Templin, E. Saltz & D. Mood. 2003. 'A model of mother-child coping and adjustment to HIV.' *Social Science and Medicine*, 56(3): 643–55.

Howarth, D. 2003. 'Discourse theory and the question of method.' Paper presented at Jesus College, Cambridge, 13 May.

Ingram, D. & S. Hutchinson. 1999. 'Defensive mothering in HIV-positive mothers.' *Qualitative Health Research*, 9(2): 243–58.

James, S. M. & P. A. Busia (eds). 1994. *Theorizing Black Feminisms: The Visionary Pragmatism of Black Women*. New York & London: Routledge.

Jeannes, L. & T. Shefer. 2004. 'Discourses of motherhood among a group of white South African mothers.' *JENdA: A Journal of Culture and African Women Studies*, 5. <http://www.jendajournal.com/issue5/jeannes.htm>.

Jones, D. J., S. R. H. Beach & R. Forehand. 2001. 'HIV infection and depressive symptoms: An investigation of African American single mothers.' *AIDS Care*, 13(3): 343–50.

Kaplan, E. A. 1992. *Motherhood and Representation: The Mother in Popular Culture and Melodrama*. London: Routledge.

Kaplan, E. A. 1994. 'Look who's talking, indeed: Fetal images in recent North American visual culture.' In E. N. Glenn, G. Chang & L. R. Forcey (eds). *Mothering: Ideology, Experience, and Agency*, pp. 121–38. New York & London: Routledge.

Kaufman, C. E. 2000. 'Reproductive control in *apartheid* South Africa.' *Population Studies*, 54(1): 105–14.

Keigher, S., B. Zabler, N. Robinson, A. Fernandez & P. E. Stevens. 2005. 'Young caregivers of mothers with HIV: Need for supports.' *Children and Youth Services Review*, 27(8): 881–904.

Kippax, S., J. Crawford, C. Waldby & P. Benton. 1990. 'Women negotiating heterosex: Implications for aids prevention.' *Women's Studies International Forum*, 13(6): 533–42.

Klein, M. 1940. 'Mourning and its relation to manic-depressive states.' Repr. in J. Mitchell (ed.). 1986. *The Selected Melanie Klein*. New York: Free Press.

Kotchick, B., R. Forehand, G. Brody & L. Armistead. 1997. 'The impact of maternal HIV infection on parenting in inner-city African American families.' *Journal of Family Psychology*, 11(4): 447–61.

Kristeva, J. 1982. *Powers of Horror: An Essay on Abjection*. Trans. L. S. Roudiez. New York: Columbia University Press.

Kristeva, J. 1986. 'Stabat mater.' In T. Moi (ed.). *The Kristeva Reader*, pp. 160–86. New York: Columbia University Press.

Kruger, L. 2003. 'Narrating motherhood: The transformative potential of individual stories.' *South African Journal of Psychology*, 33(4): 198–204.

Kruger, L. 2006. 'Motherhood.' In T. Shefer, F. Boonzaier & P. Kiguwa (eds). *The Gender of Psychology*, pp. 182–97. Cape Town: UCT Press.

Kruger, R. & G. J. Gericke. 2003. 'A qualitative exploration of rural feeding and weaning practices, knowledge and attitudes on nutrition.' *Public Health Nutrition*, 6(2): 217–23.

Landa, A. 1990. 'No accident: The voices of voluntarily childless women – An essay on the social construction of fertility choices.' In J. P. Knowles & E. Cole (eds). *Woman-defined Motherhood*, pp. 139–54. New York & London: Harrington Park Press.

Lawson, A. L. 1999. 'Women and AIDS in Africa: Sociocultural dimensions of the HIV/AIDS epidemic.' *International Social Science Journal*, 51: 391–400.

Lee, C. & R. Johann-Liang. 1999. 'Disclosure of the diagnosis of HIV/AIDS to children born of HIV-infected mothers.' *AIDS Patient Care and STDs*, 13(1): 41–45.

Lee, M. & M. Rotheram-Borus. 2001. 'Challenges associated with increased survival among parents living with HIV.' *American Journal of Public Health*, 91(8): 1303–9.

Lesch, E. & L. Kruger. 2005. 'Mothers, daughters and sexual agency in one low-income South African community.' *Social Science and Medicine*, 61: 1072–82.

Lifeline. 2004. 'Let's stop their suffering.' *Lifeline: Your News Update from the British Red Cross*, 16, Spring: 4–6.

Long, C. 2002. Finding the HIV-positive other.' *Southern African Journal of Child and Adolescent Mental Health*, 14(2): 79–90.

Long, C. 2006. 'Contradicting motherhood: HIV-positive South African mothers constructing subjectivity.' *Psychology of Women Section Review*, 8(1): 31–37.

Long, C. 2007. 'Hate in the phallic container.' *Psychoanalytic Psychotherapy in South Africa*, 15(1): 1-30.

Long, C. Forthcoming. '"I don't know who to blame": HIV-positive South African women navigating heterosexual infection.' *Psychology of Women Quarterly*.

Long, C. & E. Zietkiewicz. 2002. 'Unsettling meanings of madness: Competing constructions of South African insanity.' In D. Hook & G. Eagle (eds). *Psychopathology and Social Prejudice*, pp. 152–68. Cape Town: UCT Press.

Long, C. & E. Zietkiewicz. 2006. '"Going places": Black women negotiating race and gender in post-apartheid South Africa.' In T. Shefer, F. Boonzaier & P. Kiguwa (eds). *The Gender of Psychology*, pp. 198–219. Cape Town: UCT Press.

Lund, C. & L. Swartz. 1998. 'Xhosa-speaking schizophrenic patients' experience of their condition: Psychosis and *amafufunyana*.' *South African Journal of Psychology*, 28(2): 62–70.

Maharaj, P. 2001. 'Male attitudes to family planning in the era of HIV/AIDS: Evidence from KwaZulu-Natal, South Africa.' *Journal of Southern African Studies*, 27(2): 245–57.

Mama, A. 1995. *Beyond the Masks: Race, Gender and Subjectivity*. London & New York: Routledge.

Manopaiboon, C., N. Shaffer, L. Clark, C. Bhadrakom, W. Siriwasin, S. Chearskul, W. Suteewan, J. Kaewkungwal, A. Bennetts & T. Mastro. 1998. 'Impact of HIV on families of HIV-infected women who have recently given birth, Bangkok, Thailand.' *Journal of Acquired Immune Deficiency Syndromes and Human Retrovirology*, 18(1): 54–63.

Marcenko, M. & L. Samost. 1999. 'Living with HIV/AIDS: The voices of HIV-positive women.' *Social Work*, 44(1): 36–45.

Mariotti, P. 1997. 'Creativity and fertility: The one-parent phantasy.' In J. Raphael-Leff & R. Perelberg (eds). *Female Experience: Three Generations of British Women Psychoanalysts on Work with Women*, pp. 144–62. London: Routledge.

Marshall, H. 1991. 'The social construction of motherhood: An analysis of childcare and parenting manuals.' In A. Phoenix, A. Woollett & E. Lloyd (eds). *Motherhood: Meanings, Practices and Ideologies*, pp. 66–85. London: Sage.

Marshall, H. & A. Woollett. 2000. 'Fit to reproduce? The regulative role of pregnancy texts.' *Feminism and Psychology*, 10(3): 351–66.

McCullin, D. 2001. 'Cold heaven: Don McCullin in AIDS in Africa.' Exhibition. <http://www.christian-aid.org.uk/news/gallery/dmcullin>.

Mellins, C. A., A. A. Ehrhardt, B. Rapkin & J. F. Havens. 2000. 'Psychosocial factors associated with adaptation in HIV-infected mothers.' *AIDS and Behavior*, 4(4): 317–28.

Mendel, G. 2001. *A Broken Landscape: HIV and AIDS in Africa*. London: Blume in association with actionaid.

Mendel, G. 2002. 'Salvation is cheap.' Exhibition. <http://www.guardian.co.uk/flash/mendel.swf>.

Mendel, G. 2006. 'Looking AIDS in the face: An activist photographic project from South Africa and Mozambique.' *Virginia Quarterly Review*, 82(1):42–51.

Miles, M., P. Burchinal, D. Holditch-Davis, Y. Wasilewski & B. Christian. 1997. 'Personal, family, and health-related correlates of depressive symptoms in mothers with HIV.' *Journal of Family Psychology*, 11(1): 23–34.

Mills, M. 1997. '"The waters under the Earth": Understanding maternal depression.' In J. Raphael-Leff & R. Perelberg (eds). *Female Experience: Three Generations of British Women Psychoanalysts on Work with Women*, pp. 177–94. London: Routledge.

Mintzer, D., H. Als, E. Z. Tronick & T. B. Brazelton. 2001. 'Parenting an infant with a birth defect: The regulation of self-esteem.' In J. Raphael-Leff (ed.). *Where the Wild Things Are in Infancy and Parenting*, pp. 174–99. Colchester: Centre for Psychoanalytic Studies, University of Essex.

Mitchell, J. 1974. *Psychoanalysis and Feminism: A Radical Reassessment of Freudian Psychoanalysis*. London: Penguin.

Murphy, D. A., W. D. Marelich, M. E. Dello Stritto, D. Swendeman & A. Wiltin. 2002. 'Mothers living with HIV/AIDS: Mental, physical, and family functioning.' *AIDS Care*, 14(5): 633–44.

Murphy, L., K. Koranyi, L. Crim & S. Whited. 1999. 'Disclosure, stress and psychological adjustment among new mothers affected by HIV.' *AIDS Patient Care and STDs*, 13(2): 111–18.

Nachtwey, J. 2001. 'Death stalks a continent.' Exhibition. <http://www.time.com/time/2001/aidsinafrica/photo_flash.html>.

Naidoo, K. 2002. 'Reproductive dynamics in the context of domestic violence and economic insecurity: Findings of a South African case study.' *Journal of Asian and African Studies*, 37(3–5): 376–400.

Nhlapo, T. 1991. 'Women's rights and the family in traditional and customary law.' In S. Bazilli (ed.). *Putting Women on the Agenda*, pp. 111–23. Johannesburg: Ravan Press.

Nöstlinger, C., T. Jonckheer, E. de Belder, E. van Wijngaerden, C. Wylock, J. Pelgrom & R. Colebunders. 2004. 'Families affected by HIV: Parents' and children's characteristics and disclosure to the children.' *AIDS Care*, 16(5): 641–48.

Oakley, A. 1980. *Women Confined: Towards a Sociology of Childbirth*. Oxford: Martin Robertson.

Oakley, A. 1993. *Essays on Women, Medicine and Health*. Edinburgh: University of Edinburgh Press.

O'Barr, J. F., D. Pope & M. Wyer. 1990. 'Introduction.' In J. F. O'Barr, D. Pope & M. Wyer (eds). *Ties that Bind: Essays on Mothering and Patriarchy*, pp. 1–14. Chicago & London: University of Chicago Press.

Parker, I. 1992. *Discourse Dynamics: Critical Analysis for Social and Individual Psychology*. London: Routledge.

Parker, I. 2003. 'Psychoanalytic narratives: Writing the self into contemporary cultural phenomena.' *Narrative Inquiry*, 13(2): 301–15.

Parker, R. 1995. *Torn in Two: The Experience of Maternal Ambivalence*. London: Virago.

Patton, C. 1990. *Inventing AIDS*. London: Routledge.

Patton, C. 1993. '"With champagne and roses": Women at risk from/in AIDS discourse.' In C. Squire (ed.). *Women and AIDS: Psychological Perspectives*, pp. 165–87. London: Sage.

Patton, C. 1998. 'Women, write, AIDS.' In N. L. Roth & K. Hogan (eds). *Gendered Epidemic: Representations of Women in the Age of AIDS*, pp. ix–xiii. London: Routledge.

Peterson, N., D. Drotar, K. Olness, L. Guay & R. Kiziri-Mayengo. 2001. 'The relationship of maternal and child HIV infection to security of attachment among Ugandan infants.' *Child Psychiatry and Human Development*, 32(1): 3–17.

Phoenix, A. 1991. 'Mothers under twenty: Outsider and insider views.' In A. Phoenix, A. Woollett & E. Lloyd (eds). *Motherhood: Meanings, Practices and Ideologies*, pp. 86–102. London: Sage.

Phoenix, A., S. Frosh & R. Pattman. 2003. 'Producing contradictory masculine subject positions: Producing narratives of threat, homophobia and bullying in 11–14 year old boys.' *Journal of Social Issues*, 59: 179–95.

Phoenix, A. & A. Woollett. 1991a. 'Introduction.' In A. Phoenix, A. Woollett & E. Lloyd (eds). *Motherhood: Meanings, Practices and Ideologies*, pp. 1–12. London: Sage.

Phoenix, A. & A. Woollett. 1991b. 'Motherhood: Social construction, politics and psychology.' In A. Phoenix, A. Woollett & E. Lloyd (eds). *Motherhood: Meanings, Practices and Ideologies*, pp. 66–85. London: Sage.

Pick, W. M. & C. M. Obermeyer. 1996. 'Urbanisation, household composition and the reproductive health of women in a South African city.' *Social Science and Medicine*, 43(10): 1431–41.

Pilowsky, D., L. Wissow & N. Hutton. 2000. 'Children affected by HIV: Clinical experience and research findings.' *Child and Adolescent Psychiatric Clinics of North America*, 9(2): 451–64.

Pines, D. 1993. *A Woman's Unconscious Use of Her Body: A Psychoanalytic Perspective*. London: Virago.

Pines, D. 1997. 'The relevance of early psychic development to pregnancy and abortion.' In J. Raphael-Leff & R. Perelberg (eds). *Female Experience: Three Generations of British Women Psychoanalysts on Work with Women*, pp. 131–43. London: Routledge.

Piontelli, A. 2000 '"Is there something wrong?": The impact of technology on pregnancy.' In J. Raphael-Leff (ed.). *'Spilt Milk': Perinatal Loss and Breakdown*, pp. 39–52. London: Institute of Psychoanalysis.

Pollack, S. 1990. 'Lesbian parents: Claiming our visibility.' In J. P. Knowles & E. Cole (eds). *Woman-defined Motherhood*, pp. 181–94. New York & London: Harrington Park Press.

Potts, D. & S. Marks. 2001. 'Fertility in Southern Africa: The quiet revolution.' *Journal of Southern African Studies*, 27(2): 189–205.

Prado, G., D. J. Feaster, S. J. Schwartz, I. Abraham Pratt, L. Smith & J. Szapocznik. 2004. 'Religious involvement, coping, social support, and psychological distress in HIV-seropositive African American mothers.' *AIDS and Behavior*, 8(3): 221–35.

Raphael-Leff, J. 1991. *Psychological Processes of Childbearing*. London: Chapman & Hall.

Raphael-Leff, J. 1993. *Pregnancy: The Inside Story*. London: Sheldon.

Raphael-Leff, J. 1997. '"The casket and the key": Thoughts on creativity, gender and generative identity.' In J. Raphael-Leff & R. Perelberg (eds). *Female Experience: Three Generations of British Women Psychoanalysts on Work with Women*, pp. 237–57. London: Routledge.

Raphael-Leff, J. 2000a. 'Introduction: Technical issues in perinatal therapy.' In J. Raphael-Leff (ed.). *'Spilt Milk': Perinatal Loss and Breakdown*, pp. 7–16. London: Institute of Psychoanalysis.

Raphael-Leff, J. 2000b. '"Climbing the walls": Therapeutic intervention for post-partum disturbance.' In J. Raphael-Leff (ed.). *'Spilt Milk': Perinatal Loss and Breakdown*, pp. 60–81. London: Institute of Psychoanalysis.

Raphael-Leff, J. 2001. 'Where the wild things are.' In J. Raphael-Leff (ed.). *Where the Wild Things Are in Infancy and Parenting*, pp. 21–33. Colchester: Centre for Psychoanalytic Studies, University of Essex.

Reyland, S. A., A. Higgins-D'Alessandro & T. J. McMahon. 2002. 'Tell them you love them because you never know when things could change: Voices of adolescents living with HIV-positive mothers.' *AIDS Care*, 14(2): 285–94.

Rich, A. 1977. *Of Woman Born: Motherhood as Experience and Institution*. London: Virago.

Richardson, D. 1993. *Women, Motherhood and Childrearing*. London: Macmillan.

Robins, S. 2004. '"Long live Zackie, long live": AIDS activism, science and citizenship after apartheid.' *Journal of Southern African Studies*, 30(3): 651–72.

Rose, M. & B. Clark-Alexander. 1996. 'Coping behaviors of mothers with HIV/AIDS.' *AIDS Patient Care and STDs*, 10(1): 44–47.

Rose, N. 1989. *Governing the Soul: The Shaping of the Private Self*. London & New York: Routledge.

Rose, N. 1998. *Inventing Our Selves: Psychology, Power and Personhood*. Cambridge: Cambridge University Press.

Ross, F. 2003. *Bearing Witness: Women and the Truth and Reconciliation Commission in South Africa*. London & Sterling: Pluto Press.

Rúdólfsdóttir, A. 2000. '"I am not a patient, and I am not a child": The institutionalisation and experience of pregnancy.' *Feminism and Psychology*, 10(3): 337–50.

Sacks, V. 1996. 'Women and AIDS: An analysis of media misrepresentations.' *Social Science and Medicine*, 42(1): 59–73.

Salter Goldie, R., D. DeMatteo & S. King. 1997. 'Children born to mothers with HIV/AIDS: Family psycho-social issues.' In J. Catalán, L. Sherr & B. Hedge (eds). *The Impact of AIDS: Psychological and Social Aspects of HIV Infection*, pp. 149–58. Singapore: Harwood Academic.

Salwen, L. V. 1990. 'The myth of the wicked stepmother.' In J. P. Knowles & E. Cole (eds). *Woman-defined Motherhood*, pp. 117–26. New York & London: Harrington Park Press.

Sandelowski, M. J. 1990. 'Failures of volition: Female agency and infertility in historical perspective.' In J. O'Barr, D. Pope & M. Wyer (eds). *Ties that Bind: Essays on Mothering and Patriarchy*, pp. 35–60. Chicago & London: University of Chicago Press.

Santow, G. 1995. 'Social roles and physical health: The case of female disadvantage in poor countries.' *Social Science and Medicine*, 40(2): 147–61.

Scheper-Hughes, N. 1992. *Death without Weeping: The Violence of Everyday Life in Brazil.* Berkeley: University of California Press.

Schuster, M., M. Beckett, R. Corona & A. Zhou. 2005. 'Hugs and kisses: HIV-infected parents' fears about contagion and the effects on parent–child interaction in a nationally representative sample.' *Archives of Pediatrics and Adolescent Medicine*, 159(2): 173–79.

Seidel, G. 1990. '"Thank God I said no to AIDS": On the changing discourse of AIDS in Uganda.' *Discourse and Society*, 1(1): 61–84.

Seidel, G. 1993. 'The competing discourses of HIV/AIDS in Sub-Saharan Africa: Discourses of rights and empowerment vs. discourses of control and exclusion.' *Social Science and Medicine*, 36(3): 175–94.

Senior, L. 2002. 'Attachment theory.' In D. Hook, J. Watts & K. Cockcroft (eds). *Developmental Psychology*, pp. 247–64. Cape Town: UCT Press.

Shaffer, A., D. J. Jones, B. A. Kotchik, R. Forehand & the Family Health Project Research Group. 2001. 'Telling the children: Disclosure of maternal HIV infection and its effects on child psychosocial adjustment.' *Journal of Child and Family Studies*, 10(3): 301–13.

Shambley-Ebron, D. & J. Boyle. 2006. 'Self-care and mothering in African American women with HIV/AIDS.' *Western Journal of Nursing Research*, 28(1): 42–60.

Sherr, L. 1999. 'HIV disease and its impact on the mental health of children.' In J. Catalán (ed.). *Mental Health and HIV Infection: Psychological and Psychiatric Aspects*, pp. 42–65. London: UCL Press.

Siegel, K. & E. Gorey. 1994. 'Childhood bereavement due to parental death from acquired immunodeficiency syndrome.' *Developmental and Behavioral Pediatrics*, 15(3): S66–S70.

Silver, E. J., L. J. Baumann, S. Camacho & J. Hudis. 2003. 'Factors associated with psychological distress in urban mothers with late-stage HIV/AIDS.' *AIDS and Behavior*, 7(4): 421–31.

Simoni, J., M. Davis, J. Drossman & B. Weinberg. 2000. 'Mothers with HIV/AIDS and their children: Disclosure and guardianship issues.' *Women and Health*, 3(1): 39–54.

Sinason, V. 1992. *Mental Handicap and the Human Condition.* London: Free Association Books.

Solinger, R. 1994. 'Race and "value": Black and white illegitimate babies, 1945–1965.' In E. N. Glenn, G. Chang & L. R. Forcey (eds). *Mothering: Ideology, Experience, and Agency*, pp. 287–310. New York & London: Routledge.

Søndergaard, D. 2002. 'Theorizing subjectivity: Contesting the monopoly of psychoanalysis.' *Feminism and Psychology*, 12(4): 445–54.

Sontag, S. 1979. *On Photography*. Harmondsworth: Penguin.

Sontag, S. 1988. *AIDS and Its Metaphors*. New York: Farrar, Straus & Giroux.

Sontag, S. 2003. *Regarding the Pain of Others*. London: Hamish Hamilton.

Sprengnether, M. 1990. *The Spectral Mother: Freud, Feminism and Psychoanalysis*. Ithaca: Cornell University Press.

Squire, C. 1993. 'Introduction.' In C. Squire (ed.). *Women and AIDS: Psychological Perspectives*, pp. 1–15. London: Sage.

Squire, C. 1997. 'AIDS panic.' In J. Ussher (ed.). *Body Talk: The Material and Discursive Regulation of Sexuality, Madness and Reproduction*, pp. 50–69. London: Routledge.

Stein, A., G. Krebs, L. Richter, A. Tomkins, T. Rochat & M. Bennish. 2005. 'Babies of the pandemic.' *Archives of Disease in Childhood*, 90: 116–18.

Steiner, D. 1997. 'Mutual admiration between mother and baby: A *folie à deux*?' In J. Raphael-Leff & R. Perelberg (eds). *Female Experience: Three Generations of British Women Psychoanalysts on Work with Women*, pp. 163–76. London: Routledge.

Stern, D. 1995. *The Motherhood Constellation*. London: Basic Books.

Stimmel, B. 2004. 'The cause is worse: Remeeting Jocasta.' *International Journal of Psychoanalysis*, 85: 1175–89.

Strebel, A. 1992. '"There's absolutely nothing I can do, just believe in God": South African women with AIDS.' *Agenda*, 12: 50–62.

Strebel, A. 1997. 'Putting discourse analysis to work in AIDS prevention.' In A. Levett, A. Kottler, E. Burman & I. Parker (eds). *Culture, Power and Difference: Discourse Analysis in South Africa*, pp. 109–21. London: Zed Books.

Surrey, J. L. 1990. 'Mother-blaming and clinical theory.' In J. P. Knowles & E. Cole (eds). *Woman-defined Motherhood*, pp. 83–88. New York & London: Harrington Park Press.

Swartz, L. 1998. *Thinking about Culture and Mental Health: A Southern African View*. Cape Town: Oxford University Press.

TAC (Treatment Action Campaign). 2004. *TAC Electronic Newsletter*. 3 December. <http://www.tac.org.za/newsletter/2004/ns03_12_2004.htm>.

TAC (Treatment Action Campaign). 2008. Website. <http://www.tac.org.za/community/keystatistics>.

Taylor, E., N. Amodei & R. Mangos. 1996. 'The presence of psychiatric disorders in HIV-infected women.' *Journal of Counselling Development*, 74: 345–51.

Taylor, S. 2001. 'Evaluating and applying discourse analytic research.' In M. Wetherell, S. Taylor & S. J. Yates (eds). *Discourse as Data: A Guide for Analysis*, pp. 311–29. London: Sage in association with the Open University.

Thairu, L. N., G. H. Pelto, N. C., Rollins, R. M. Bland & N. Ntshangase. 2005. 'Sociocultural influences on infant feeding decisions among HIV-infected women in rural Kwa-Zulu Natal, South Africa.' *Maternal and Child Nutrition*, 1(1): 2–10.

Tomlinson, M., P. Cooper & L. Murray. 2005. 'The mother–infant relationship and infant attachment in a South African peri-urban settlement.' *Child Development*, 76(5): 1044–54.

Treichler, P. 1988. 'AIDS, homophobia, and biomedical discourse: An epidemic of signification.' In D. Crimp (ed.). *AIDS: Cultural Analysis/Cultural Activism*, pp. 31–70. Cambridge, Mass.: MIT Press.

UNAIDS (Joint UN Action Plan on HIV/AIDS). 2004. *AIDS Epidemic Update*. <http://www.unaids.org/wad2004/report.html>.

UNAIDS (Joint UN Action Plan on HIV/AIDS). 2008. *2008 Report on the Global AIDS Epidemic*. <http://www.unaids.org/en/KnowledgeCentre/HIVData/GlobalReport/2008/2008_Global.report.asp>.

Upton, R. L. 2001. '"Infertility makes you invisible": Gender, health and the negotiation of fertility in northern Botswana.' *Journal of Southern African Studies*, 27(2): 349–62.

Ussher, J. 1989. *The Psychology of the Female Body*. London: Routledge.

Van Loon, R. 2000. 'Redefining motherhood: Adaptation to role change for women with AIDS.' *Families in Societies: The Journal of Contemporary Human Services*, 81(2): 152–61.

Venuti, L. 1992. *Rethinking Translation: Discourse, Subjectivity, Ideology*. London & New York: Routledge.

Walker, C. 1982. *Women and Resistance in South Africa*. London: Onyx Press.

Walker, C. 1990. 'Women and gender in Southern Africa to 1945: An overview.' In C. Walker (ed.). *Women and Gender in Southern Africa to 1945*, pp. 1–32. Cape Town: David Philip.

Walker, C. 1991. *Women and Resistance in South Africa*, 2nd ed. Cape Town & Johannesburg: David Philip; New York: Monthly Review Press.

Walker, C. 1995. 'Conceptualising motherhood in twentieth century South Africa.' *Journal of Southern African Studies*, 21(3): 417–37.

Walker, L., G. Reid & M. Cornell. 2004. *Waiting to Happen: HIV/AIDS in South Africa – The Bigger Picture*. Colorado & London: Lynne Rienner; Cape Town: Double Storey Books.

Walkerdine, V. 1984. 'Developmental psychology and the child-centred pedagogy: The insertion of Piaget into early education.' In J. Henriques, W. Hollway, C. Urwin, C. Venn & V. Walkerdine (eds). *Changing the Subject: Psychology, Social Regulation and Subjectivity*, pp. 153–202. London & New York: Methuen.

Walkerdine, V., H. Lucey & J. Melody. 2001. *Growing up Girl: Psychosocial Explorations of Gender and Class*. Basingstoke: Palgrave.

Warner, M. 1976. *Alone of All Her Sex: The Myth and the Cult of the Virgin Mary*. London: Weidenfeld & Nicolson.

Warner, M. 1985. *Monuments and Maidens: The Allegory of the Female Form*. Berkeley & Los Angeles: University of California Press.

Warner, M. 1994. *Six Myths of Our Time: Managing Monsters*. The Reith Lectures 1994. London: Vintage.

Wegar, K. 1997. 'In search of bad mothers: Social constructions of birth and adoptive motherhood.' *Women's Studies International Forum*, 20(1): 77–86.

Welldon, E. 1988. *Mother, Madonna, Whore: The Idealization and Denigration of Motherhood*. London: Free Association Books.

Wetherell, M. 1999. 'Discursive psychology and psychoanalysis: Theorising masculine subjectivities.' Paper presented at the Millennium World Conference of Critical Psychology, University of Western Sydney, 30 April–2 May.

Wetherell, M. 2002. 'Assessing the place of culture in social thought.' Paper presented at the Pavis Centre conference on Cultural Returns, Oxford, September.

Wetherell, M. 2005. 'Unconscious conflict or everyday accountability? A commentary on Hollway and Jefferson.' *British Journal of Social Psychology*, 44(2): 169–73.

Willig, C. 2000. 'A discourse-dynamic approach to the study of subjectivity in health psychology.' *Theory and Psychology*, 10(4): 547–70.

Winnicott, D. 1964. *The Child, the Family and the Outside World.* Harmondsworth: Pelican.

Winnicott, D. 1971. *Playing and Reality.* Hove & New York: Brunner-Routledge.

Winnicott, D. 1987. 'Hate in the countertransference.' In *Through Paediatrics to Psycho-Analysis,* pp. 194–203. London: Hogarth Press & Institute of Psycho-Analysis. Originally published 1947.

Woodward, K. 1997. 'Motherhood: Identities, meanings and myths.' In K. Woodward (ed.). *Identity and Difference,* pp. 239–98. London: Sage in association with the Open University.

Woollett, A. & A. Phoenix. 1991. 'Psychological views of mothering.' In A. Phoenix, A. Woollett & E. Lloyd (eds). *Motherhood: Meanings, Practices and Ideologies,* pp. 66–85. London: Sage.

Young, I. 1990. 'Pregnant embodiment: Subjectivity and alienation.' *Journal of Medicine and Philosophy,* 9: 45–62.

Zivi, K. 1998. 'Constituting the "clean and proper" body: Convergences between abjection and AIDS.' In N. L. Roth & K. Hogan (eds). *Gendered Epidemic: Representations of Women in the Age of AIDS,* pp. 33–63. London: Routledge.

Index

abortion 159-160, 204
adoption 39, 61-62, 157-159, 204
'African AIDS' 25-26
Afrikaner nationalism, see apartheid
AIDS myths in South Africa 47-49
antiretrovirals, see Nevirapine
antiretrovirals
apartheid 76-78
    black fears associated with family
        planning 78
    family planning 78
attachment 93-94, 139, 142, 200
    bad 202

baby
    all important 3, 22, 105, 171, 187
    as cure, saviour 164-165
    good and innocent 170
    power of body 205
    subject of social discourses 198
breastfeeding vs bottle feeding 17, 37-38,
    52, 136, 137-141, 160, 162, 200, 204

caesarean section 125
childbirth/childbearing
    fear of 67
    medicalisation of 59-60
    process 153-154
childcare manuals 58, 60, 61
Christianity 43, 47, 48, 76, 88
clinics
    antenatal 31
    context 29
    frequency 30
    postnatal 31-32
    therapies available 30-31
    women's attendance at 32, 34
colonialism 76, 78
condoms 31, 33, 39-40, 47, 51, 78, 130

discourse
    AIDS 25, 47, 52-53
    application in this book 101-102,
        104
    definition of 99-100
    discourse analysis/theory 5, 96, 99-
        104
    post-modern approach 99, 100
    power of 157-60, 166, 169, 176,
        192-193
    psychoanalytical approach 5, 96-104
    subjectivity 100, 102-104, 196
domestic violence 39, 80

extended family, role of 182-183

family values 36, 37, 40-41, 44
fertility 76, 78, 79
Foucault, M. 59-60, 103

gender 5, 18, 24, 34, 47, 51, 53, 56, 63, 65,
    76, 77, 78, 99, 103-104, 106, 147, 151, 195
grandmother 12

HIV
    diagnosis 1-2, 24, 44-45, 51, 84-86,
        88, 90, 91, 94, 97, 114, 118, 121-123,
        125, 131, 177-178, 180, 202
    disclosure of 28, 30-31, 45, 46, 83,
        84-85
    myths 47-48
    prevalence/rates/statistics 1, 28, 82
    stigma/discrimination/prejudice 4,
        23, 41-42, 43, 46, 53, 177
    tests, fear of 122-123
    transmission 3, 42, 44, 106
HIV-negative 10, 15, 33, 37, 43, 45, 46,
    50, 51, 52, 86, 90, 91, 93, 94, 106, 109,
    112, 114-115, 118, 121-124, 129, 133-135,
    161-162, 164-165, 178-180, 199

HIV-positive motherhood (*see also*
maternal, mother, motherhood)
ambivalence, anger/fear 173-177
conceptions of future 3, 84, 88, 92,
106, 110, 190, 199
desires 5, 45, 70. 98, 134, 143-144,
157, 159, 164, 171-172, 173,
180, 183, 185, 192, 194, 195,
197, 198, 202, 205, 207
fear/fears 3, 18, 32, 37, 39, 42, 45-46, 49,
51, 78, 80, 83, 84, 91-92, 98, 110,
119, 120, 125, 128-129, 132, 134,
135, 136, 139-140, 143, 150, 151,
153, 155, 161, 162, 164, 173, 175,
176, 177, 181, 183, 185, 189, 195,
199, 200, 201, 202, 203, 204, 206
guilt 10, 18, 21, 49, 64, 70-71,
83-85, 88, 95, 98, 110, 121, 132,
134, 136-138, 141-143, 152,
160, 161, 165-166, 173, 176,
178, 191, 199-200, 205, 206
images of 190-192
in South Africa 1, 8, 24, 27, 28, 44,
53, 93, 124
lack of literature/research on 3-4,
83, 92
pregnancy 27, 30-31, 42, 59, 106,
109, 110, 112
psychiatric symptoms of 85-87
shame 10, 87, 120, 159
husband, *see* male partners

infertility 79-80
infertility in Africa 79-80
intergenerational aspects of HIV
motherhood 181-182
interviewees
attitude to interviewer 33-34
Amara 110, 112, 117, 129, 186
Anele 157-160, 186-187
Ayanda 116-117, 134-136, 153-154,
156-157, 174-175, 186
Boitumelo 122-123, 136-137
Bongiwe 148-152, 203
Charity 108-110
Dikeledi 115-116, 118, 129, 132-134, 139

Hlengiwe 35-39, 118-119, 175, 184
introduction/overview 23-27
Joyce 112, 137, 181-182
Khanya 165-166
Kuli 113, 129
Leleti 43-46, 171-172, 187
Lesedi 129, 164-165, 175
Lukanyo 119-120, 129-132, 134,
138, 160-161, 163-164
Lungile 141, 153, 172
Mandisa 113-115, 121, 154
Neo 110-112, 144, 183
Nombeko 46-51, 146-147, 173-176
Nonyameko 107, 121-122, 177-180
Palesa 123
Petunia 137-138, 171
Phindiwe 161-162
Pumla 39-43
Thandiwe 110, 119, 139, 152-153,
172-173, 185-186
Tumi 140, 154-155
Zinzi 140-141, 165
Zodwa 107, 138
interviews
categories of women 4
comparison with photographs 23,
191
content 4, 208
language used 28-29
number of 4, 29
setting 27, 29
interviewer's HIV status 33

Jocasta's tale (*see also* motherhood,
psychoanalytic approach to) 63-65, 71
Joseph 12

male partners 12, 28, 35-36, 39-40, 41,
44, 49, 51, 61, 86, 93, 130-131, 143,
151, 157, 161, 177-178, 180, 203
maternal (*see also* mother, motherhood)
ambivalence/ambiguity 69-71, 166,
173-74, 176-77, 203, 206
attentiveness 185-186, 199
body as creative/destructive,
nourishing/threatening 60, 166

body, power of 203
care 22, 30, 95, 108, 109, 119,
    127-129, 133-134,142, 145,
    154-155, 171, 182, 185, 186,
    190, 194, 199, 201
desires 64-66, 162, 181, 202
fear 2, 27, 148, 152-153, 169, 171,
observation 107, 112-113, 118, 123,
    124, 127, 129, 164, 165-166,
    194, 197
selflessness 54-55, 58, 66, 75, 105,
    143, 158-159, 170, 173, 177,
    185, 195, 203, 204
subjectivity 4, 22, 57, 60-74, 128,
    143, 146, 155, 156, 159, 163,
    167, 168-169, 170, 188, 194,
    196-197, 202-203, 205, 207
Mendel, Gideon photo essay in *The
    Guardian* 8-11, 14-18
mother (*see also* maternal)
position of absence 146, 169
unimportant 3-4, 22, 105
Western mothers focused on in
    literature 25-26, 62, 98
motherhood (*see also* maternal)
African motherhood 78-80
deconstruction of 55-57, 62
developmental theory of 66-67
fantasy/fantasies 3, 58, 63, 65, 66-67,
    97, 98, 102, 104, 111, 150-151,
    160, 164-166, 173, 176, 178-180,
    191, 197
feminist approach to 63, 72-75, 80
good mother/bad mother 58-59,
    61-62, 71, 96-97, 161-162, 166,
    172-173, 200-201, 204
idealisation and denigration of 57-58,
    68, 71, 73, 80
in South Africa 75-80
Placental Paradigm 68-69
projection 68, 70, 98-99, 177, 191
psychoanalytic approach to 63-75,
    80, 96-98, 104
splits/splitting in perception of 1,
    26, 68, 69-72, 98, 146, 156, 162,
    188, 192, 195, 197, 204, 207

theory and discourse of 3, 6, 55-63,
    99-104
Western attitude to 46, 76, 80, 182,
mother-infant interaction (*see also*
    maternal) 201-202
early mother-infant attachment 93-94,
    127-144
Mother Theresa 58

Nachtwey, James, photo essay in *Time*,
    10, 12-13
Nevirapine/antiretrovirals 2, 29- 31, 37,
    48, 106, 118-20, 148
cost of treatment 30
treatment 29-30

photographs of HIV-positive motherhood
    5-6, 7, 8-9, 11-12, 13-18, 82
post-colonial Africa, Western images of
    6-7
power/powerlessness 39, 40, 56-57, 60,
    71, 76, 97, 102, 103-104, 138, 152,
    166, 190, 192, 193, 198
power relations 5, 24, 56, 63, 97, 99-100
pregnancy, psychodynamic theories of
    66, 147-148

race 24, 32, 34, 47, 53, 76, 99, 104

slips in literature 83
Sontag, Susan 6-8

traditional healers/medicine/practices
    48-49

urbanisation/urban-rural divide 34, 46,
    75-78, 182

viral load 178
Virgin Mary 2, 12, 57

Zionist Christian Church (ZCC) 47

Printed and bound by CPI Group (UK) Ltd, Croydon, CR0 4YY

09/06/2025

14685816-0002

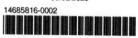